Fit Happens!
Simple Steps for a Healthier,
More Productive Life!

Be Well!

Todd Whitthorne

Fit Happens!
Simple Steps for a Healthier, More Productive Life!

Todd Whitthorne

First published by Dog Ear Publishing
4011 Vincennes Rd
Indianapolis, IN 46268
www.dogearpublishing.net

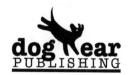

ISBN: 978-1-4575-6132-0

This book is printed on acid-free paper.

Printed in the United States of America

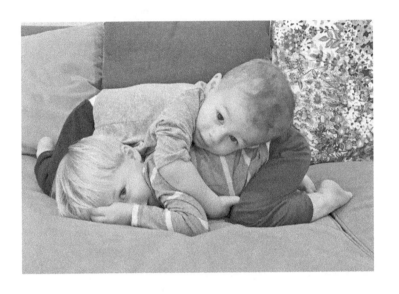

To Henry and Hudson…no offense dudes,
but I don't want to *watch* you play.
However, I fully intend to play *with you* for a long, long time!

I love you!
Pops

Good health is not about temporary behavior change.
It's about building healthy habits that will last a lifetime!

- TW

Contents

Part 3. Looking Downfield

Foreword

In the late summer of 2010, while returning from a Canadian fishing vacation with my family, I found myself most uneasy while staring out the window from the passenger's seat of my brother's large SUV, which was rumbling south on a stretch of interstate somewhere between Kenora, Ontario and Maple Grove, Minnesota. The trees zipped by in a shifting, blurry mélange and the accompanying soundtrack was the shrieking chatter of his kids and mine. My dad was in the backseat and in his familiar posture with headphones on, listening to a book on tape, while deftly paging through a stack of legal documents.

Something happened to me that day, but it had been building I suppose for years and years. What I remember is that in a single instant, while staring out the window, I experienced an unprecedented wave of anxiety and terror that consumed my body, overtook my mind, and rattled my soul. The journey out of the depths of that pit to simply being functional took months and began later that day with a series of phone calls to a very few people I trusted.

One of the first calls was to Todd Whitthorne.

I don't remember when we met for the first time exactly but Whit and I became fast friends. I'm pulled like a magnet to smart, funny, gregarious and talented. And if either of us said that aloud to the other – we would immediately follow it up with – "and so I must ask myself why the hell am I spending any time with YOU?" - or something deprecating like that.

But on this phone call – the first in what would become hundreds over the next few months for Whit, and me, the playful exchanges gave way to somber discussion and serious problem solving. I was in crisis, and Whit helped dig me out and quite honestly, he helped save my life.

It was hardly my first bout with my demons. They were first formally confronted in May of 1986 while I was a patient at Hazelden Treatment Center for drug and alcohol abuse, and at subsequent countless counseling and therapy sessions and twelve-step meetings. I read books, gave speeches, sought information, and shared openly. I walked the walk. The thing about demons though, they don't go away so easily. You think you got 'em licked but they're always hanging around. Demons are patient. Demons play the long game. And when they see an opening, they strike hard.

My job in those days was as the play-by-play TV and radio broadcaster for the Dallas Stars hockey team, and I was concerned about whether or not I'd be able to get myself on the air and performing just a few weeks later. I was married and had a teenage daughter and I had obligations to them too. And I was afraid to leave the house.

Whit helped organize doctors and comprehensive physical and mental well-being checkups, and found me a therapist. All of these things were helpful and necessary. I had help from others too to locate resources and people and programs and I worked to attack them with the same kind of tenacity I bring to everything in my life, albeit at the time, mitigated by anxiety-induced paralysis. Little by little, phone call by phone call, appointment by appointment, I found strength to leave the house. But I had lost weight, was smoking about a pack a day, and was on very shaky ground. Every day I woke up wondering if I would in fact make it through the day. Whit was there for all of it. He was always available by phone, and marshaled his considerable network of health professionals to work with me.

The best and longest lasting contribution Whit made to my general wellbeing and the quality of life I enjoy today however started out as a fairly innocuous invitation one day to join him for a bike ride.

I said – "Whit – man – I haven't been on a bike in years…"

To which he responded – "don't worry – it's just like riding a bike…"

I thought – oh what the hell. At that point, I would have tried anything. I didn't own a bike so I went to the bike shop and purchased one. It was a good starter bike and he kept the pace slow and easy for the first ride. Bicycles are wonderful contraptions and getting on one again I was quite literally taken on a journey back through the careless days of my youth. Try it sometime if you haven't in a long time. You'll see what I mean.

"Ok – next Saturday morning same time then." Whit declared at the end of that first ride.

"Ok."

Over the course of several morning rides I started feeling a little better. The therapy helped, the meds helped, meditating helped, but dang man – the bike rides! A couple hours every Saturday morning on a bike with frequent stops to talk and reflect. The first few rides the conversation was about how I was doing, but that subject got pushed aside and we started having more ordinary conversations. At Whit's urging I was becoming more like myself again. But – a better and more lasting version of myself.

Whit started talking to me about vitamins and supplements and better nutrition and I started paying attention. I began eating better, taking fewer meds, sleeping better. Whit's knowledge and approach is simply unique. He practices what he preaches and is the living embodiment of someone who takes his own advice. Without Whit – I don't know where I would have wound up.

I made it on the air for opening night and every night thereafter. My colleagues at work made allowances for me, and for that I'll always be grateful. They too helped carry me when I couldn't completely carry myself.

I quit smoking a few months later. Finally. I made connections between my body and my mind and my soul. It was hard work. It was excruciating. But I worked hard and got myself back on track. And it's not something I did for a short time and am done with. My life has changed.

These days, I exercise regularly. I do cardio boxing, a little running, weight lifting, and yes, cycling – on a better bike. Some days I can even overtake Whit on the uphill runs. Those are really good days… I watch what I eat. I take vitamins and supplements. I'm 56 years old and am in the best physical shape of my life. Turns out my head's in a good spot too.

The demons are still there I should think. Waiting. Hoping for a misstep or a crack. But they're less likely to find any.

I know that when you read this book you'll gain great insight and get usable tools to integrate into your own life to help you live your best life possible. I know you'll enjoy reading what's ahead.

But now – I gotta go – I gotta call Whit and set up our next ride.

Ralph Strangis

Preface

The first step is to establish that something is possible;
then probability will occur.
—Elon Musk, founder of Tesla and co-founder of PayPal

I've worked in the wellness space since the late 1990s. As president of a health consulting firm, I guide product development, marketing and sales, and client consulting strategies in health and corporate wellness. Before that, I spent more than a decade assisting organizations in developing strategies to increase employee health and productivity and to decrease healthcare-related costs. I also directed an in-residence behavior-modification program and a nutritional supplement line. I am passionate about helping individuals improve their quality of life. As a health and wellness speaker, I've worked with hundreds of organizations looking to boost healthy living, fitness, and corporate wellness.

The simple fact that you are reading this book most likely indicates that you are searching for a way to feel better. Individuals state their goals in a variety of ways: "I wish I had more energy"; "I want to lose weight"; "My wife is worried that I'm not taking care of myself"; "I need to lower my blood pressure"; "My doctor has told me if I don't improve my health, I'll never be able to get pregnant"; "My daughter is getting married soon, and I don't want to embarrass her when I walk down the aisle." There are all sorts of reasons, but once you really boil it down—when you peel back the layers of the onion, so to speak—what folks are looking for is simply to *feel* better.

Would *you* like to feel better? You can! There is absolutely no debate; I guarantee it: It's possible. I see it regularly, almost daily, in individuals who had basically given up, convinced there was no way on earth they could ever gain control of their life. That was then; now they are living radically different lives. They look better, sleep better, work better, love better, and are better parents and spouses, all because they *feel* better, both physically and emotionally.

Don't get me wrong; I'm not saying it's easy. I'm saying it's *possible*. No doubt about it: Embracing healthy behaviors positively influences all areas of performance, both personally and professionally. What it requires is *change,* and for some people, change is really hard, especially in today's obesogenic environment. But as the late great motivational speaker Zig Ziglar pointed out, "If you keep doing what you've been doing, then you'll keep getting what you've been getting." The absolute fundamental, cast-in-stone, nonnegotiable, underlying common theme for success for anyone is this: When the student is ready, the teacher will appear! This is vitally important, so I'll say it again: When the student is ready, the teacher will appear. Simply put: If you're not ready to change your life, you won't.

There are more than seven and a half billion people in the world, but no one has more impact on your health and well-being than you do. No one! Not your doctor, not your employer, not your spouse, and certainly not the government. I encourage you to ask yourself two questions: *What* do you really want, and *why* do you want it? If you're honest with yourself, your true motivation is probably much more significant than just the number on the scale. Your weight is an important component of health and certainly plays a role in how you feel and function, but if you define yourself solely by what you weigh, it's going to be very hard for you to have long-term success.

It's important to define *why* improving your health is important to you. If you are motivated merely because someone has nagged you so much that you've finally agreed to change just to shut them up, odds are that your motivation is not going to last very long. It's okay to be selfish about your health; in fact, it's mandatory, because if you don't take proper care of yourself, it'll be extremely hard for you to effectively care for others.

I'm delighted you've made it this far. If you are ready for change, to become the healthy, happy, productive person you envision yourself being—and that you were designed to be—I'm ready to help you get there.

In three parts, this book offers simple steps on healthy living. Part 1, "Getting Real," defines the challenges inherent in today's hyper-challenging environment; the ways we eat, work, and live are fast-tracking many Americans to poor health. Knowing your risk factors is key to getting real and committing to invest in yourself. Part 2, "Embracing Healthy Behaviors," provides specifics on the benefits of solid nutrition and regular exercise, explains how weight loss actually works, and debunks a few myths along the way.

Once you know *what* to do, how do you *keep* doing it? Part 3, "Looking Downfield," helps you find sustaining motivation, allowing you to go beyond the basics to build the habit of everyday excellence. With a commitment to lifelong healthy behaviors, you can achieve better performance in all areas of your life.

Be patient with yourself, have some faith in this guide, and let your body and your mind amaze you. Fit happens!

Let's get to work!

*Author's Note - As you will soon see, this book is filled with inspirational quotes from a variety of individuals; some famous, some not. Whenever possible, I have attributed the quotes to their original source. If you are interested, the quotes are also listed together in this book starting on page 171.

ACKNOWLEDGMENTS

I've been amazingly blessed to be inspired, taught, and mentored by some incredible individuals throughout my life. Fortunately, many of them have become close friends and this book would have never come to be without their encouragement, input, and support.

From 2000 to 2007, I hosted and produced a nationally syndicated radio program called *Healthy Living* with Dr. Ken Cooper, who is often referred to as the "Father of Aerobics." When Dr. Cooper was not available for the broadcast I had the chance to reach out to experts from all over the country and help share their vast knowledge with the listeners. I was in constant search of what I called, "Switzerlands"— individuals who did not have a product to push or an axe to grind, just really smart folks dedicated to finding ways to help us all live better lives. It was an amazing opportunity for me to build a contact base of health experts who played a major role in the inspiration of this book. My sincere thanks go to Dr. Joseph Hibbeln, Dr. Bill Harris, Dr. Robert Abel, Dr. Pat Fulgham, Dr. Jorn Dyerberg, Dr. Craig Schwimmer, the late Phil Lawler, Dr. Miriam Nelson, Dr. David Katz and, of course, Dr. Cooper.

My tenure with the Cooper organization began in 1999 and totaled 14 years. The list of former colleagues who somehow contributed to this book is a long one and includes Dr. Tedd Mitchell and his wife, Dr. Janet Tornelli-Mitchell, Dr. Steven Blair, Dr. Charles Sterling, Dr. Cameron Nelson, Dr. John Cannaday, Dr. Michele Kettles, Dr. Abram Eisenstein, Dr. Riva Rahl, Dr. Chris Abel, Rob Nelson, Kathy Duran-Thal, RDN, Jennifer Neily, RDN, Patty Kirk, RDN, Kathy Miller, RDN, Meridan Zerner, RDN, Clayton Arhelger, Connie Tyne, Susie Kania, Cindy Bostick, Cathy Sides, Erika Jefferson, Dr. Susan Campbell, Deb Hanry and the late, great Fred Meyer.

Other friends and colleagues in the scientific and health community that I'm greatly appreciative of include Dr. Eduardo Sanchez, Dr. Kevin Gilliland, Dr. Conrad Earnest, Gordie Echtenkamp, David Michel, Pete Egoscue, Dr. Baker Harrell, Becky Brosche, Marcia Upson, Dr. Dana Labat, Doug Cropper, J.C. Montgomery, Robert Walker, Dr. Donald Fischer, Dr. Catrine Tudor-Locke, Dwight Mankin, Ted Borgstadt, Crayton Webb, Betty Garrett, Gail Davis, Julie and Bob Benson, Dr. Tom Geppert, Dave Muscari, Kevin Bingham, Doug Gaynor, and Mark Everest.

My personal goal of "leaving the campground cleaner than I found it" has, in large part, been made possible by my decision to join ACAP Health in 2013. The incredible team that I'm fortunate to work with on a daily basis makes what I do for a living amazingly satisfying. To all of the "A-Team" I offer a sincere THANK YOU! It's an honor for me to work with every one of you. Two leaders who deserve a dedicated shout-out are Den Bishop and Wally Gomaa, who were instrumental in helping me see the massive impact that we could make in improving the health of thousands, and soon millions, of Americans.

I would particularly like to recognize and thank my great friend and colleague, Dr. Tim Church. Tim has been instrumental in helping open my mind to the importance of public health, which he likes to describe as "doing the most good for the most people." Not only is Tim highly credentialed, holding an MD, PhD, and an MPH, he has constantly encouraged me to "look downfield." Our constant interaction since we first met in 1999 has indelibly shaped the way I think about and communicate the importance of health. Thank you, my brother!

Speaking of brothers, as the only child of only children, close friendships have always been a priority of mine. I'm extremely grateful for the very tight circle of "my brothers," many of which I've known since elementary school. I'm honored to have shared my life with Chris Lagudis (kindergarten), Sam White (first grade),

John Klimmek (third grade), Scott McClelland (sixth grade), Rex Bein, Geoff Yates, Rick DeGabrielle, Rick Dillon, and Glenn Griggs. I also am amazingly thankful for the positive influence that Chris' parents, Steve and Susie Lagudis, continue to have on me.

While I've been working on *Fit Happens!* for over a decade, it took a small team of true professionals to help me get the book across the goal line. My sincere thanks to my editor, Amy Smith-Bell, for her patience, guidance, and literary expertise. Amy, you were terrific to work with! A great deal of credit also goes to Adrienne Miller and Stephanie Stringham from Dog Ear Publishing for their assistance in putting the final bow on the project. In addition, huge props to my colleague, Brett White, since without his effort, this dude would have never found the end zone! A special shout-out to Michael Ernst and Blake White for taking many of the terrific photographs on our trek up Mt. Kilimanjaro. Thanks also to my buddy, Ralph Strangis, for not only writing the forward, but for being so transparent. I hope your message serves as an inspiration to others.

Last, but certainly not least, I want to thank my family for always supporting my passion for health. I know my enthusiasm can sometimes be a bit extreme, so to my wife, Kathy, daughter, Lauren, son-in-law, Scott, and son, Andrew — thank you for allowing me to share the excitement I have for trying to make a difference. I love you all very much!

PART 1

Getting Real

"You can't live a perfect day without doing something for someone who will never be able to repay you."
– John Wooden

1.

A Cleaner Campground:
Success versus Significance

When I was a young boy growing up in Southern California, before team sports started dominating my time and attention, I was a Cub Scout. Two or three times a year, we would go camping, often in the San Bernardino Mountains. Those experiences are some of my fondest memories. Mr. George Bein, one of my Scout leaders, was a large, stern German man who always said the same thing when we finished setting up our tents: "Men, remember, we need to leave the campground cleaner than we found it." Although I am still friends with Mr. Bein's son Rex, I'm sorry I never took the opportunity to thank his dad. Mr. Bein's edict became my metaphor for life.

I believe we are all on this earth for a reason: to have a positive impact on the lives of others. Each of us is not an island. Rather, life is a team sport, and to make a measurable impact—to leave a clean campground—we all need to take care of ourselves. It seems a bit counterintuitive, but to positively influence those around us, we have to become a bit selfish. We have to invest in ourselves to become strong and healthy enough to make a difference.

The human body is beautifully designed and will do exactly what we ask it to do, both good and bad. Treat it well with regular exercise, healthful food, and plenty of sleep, and the body will respond in amazing ways. Conversely, if we refuse to engage in physical activity, eat nothing but junk, abuse alcohol and tobacco, and routinely try to operate without much sleep, then the body, and overall health, will suffer—maybe not right away, but it's only a matter of time.

All of us, if we think about it, are in a position to have a positive influence on someone else: a child, spouse, friend, neighbor, or colleague. Or perhaps we can affect a large group or organization, such as a classroom or school, church, club, team, or business. If we really want to make a difference, we need all the energy and stamina we can get; it's extremely difficult to influence anything or anybody if we hurt all the time or if we're sad or depressed. Think about the differences we can make when we feel great and when our outlooks are positive. Each of us is in charge of cultivating this outlook for ourselves; no one else is.

Social entrepreneur Bob Buford wrote a book in 2008 titled *Halftime: Moving from Success to Significance.* The primary theme was that many of us spend our early adult years—the twenties, thirties, and forties—laser-focused on acquiring typical markers of "success": job, salary, title, house, car, etc. Once we obtain these things, however, we realize that achieving these milestones is not all that satisfying, and we experience a rather empty feeling. You might remember the old Peggy Lee song "Is That All There Is?" I certainly believe in working hard to support ourselves and our families, but I also believe that we have a higher calling. Each of us has been given a wonderful body and mind, with amazing potential. We need to appreciate these gifts and develop a game plan to maximize our health.

We all have the capability to do something *significant*, to positively affect the lives of others and to leave the campground cleaner than we found it. Strive for significance!

> "Take the first step in faith. You don't have to see the whole staircase, just take the first step."
> – Dr. Martin Luther King

"Knowing is not enough; we must apply.
Wishing is not enough; we must do."
– Johann Van Goethe

2.

The Way We Eat, Work, and Live: Today's Obesogenic Environment

As humans, we are rather myopic; sometimes we believe that history began the year we were born. But the world we live in today is way different than it was fifty or a hundred years ago, and even, in some cases, just five years ago. The way most Americans live is not the way we were designed to live. In the 1950s, there were 2,000 food items in a grocery store; in the 1960s, 5,000 food items; and today, in a big-box grocery store, there are 60,000 to 70,000 food items available! Notice I didn't say "foods" but "food items." Most of the offerings on grocery shelves are what best-selling food writer Michael Pollan has referred to as "man-made food-like substances"—combinations of ingredients (often fat, sugar, and salt) engineered along with a plethora of chemicals and artificial flavors and scents, designed to activate the human brain and drive craveability. The result? Sadly, since the late 1970s, the U.S. obesity rate for adults has nearly tripled. As of 2017, almost 4 in 10 Americans are obese (39.6 percent). The childhood obesity rate has now hit 18.5 percent!

How We Eat: Big Food Companies

If you're older than thirty-five, you'll be able to complete this jingle, even though you probably haven't heard it in years. Here goes: "Two all-beef patties . . ." That's it, you've got it. Isn't that amazing? For younger readers, let me explain: In 1968,

McDonald's introduced the Big Mac nationally. In 1974, it launched a massive ad campaign that included this catchy jingle: "Two all-beef patties, special sauce, lettuce, cheese, pickles, onions—on a sesame-seed bun." At many of the McDonald's franchises, if you went to the counter and recited the jingle in a certain amount of time, usually two to three seconds, you would be rewarded a free Big Mac.

What a brilliant idea! This was my first exposure to drug-dealer marketing: "Hey, kid, try this . . . the first one is free; after that, ya gotta pay!" And man, are we paying! The processed-food industry in the United States accounts for one trillion dollars a year in sales. The big food companies spend millions of dollars promoting foods and drinks that are cheap, convenient, and chemically engineered to taste fantastic. The average American now eats thirty-three pounds of cheese per year (triple what we ate in 1970). (Cheese, by the way, contains high levels of saturated fat.) Each of us, on average, ingests close to one hundred pounds of sugar, compared to 6.2 pounds per person per year in 1822. Oh, and don't forget the salt. We down about 3,400 milligrams of salt per day (the recommended daily intake for anyone four or older, based on a 2,000-calorie diet, is no more than 2,300 milligrams per day, and for certain groups is limited to 1,500 milligrams per day). Of interest is that salt comes mostly in processed foods (canned soups and salty snack foods like chips and crackers) rather than from the shaker on the table.

This is quite a contrast to "the good old days," when your great-grandmother would go out back, pick some fruits and vegetables from her garden, grab a chicken, wring its neck, and make supper (what we now call dinner). There was no fast-food drive-thrus, frozen dinners, Domino's pizza-delivery options, store-bought Lunchables for school days, or triple-mocha Frappuccinos with "extra whip" available on every street corner, 24/7. No refillable Big Gulps, all-you-can-eat buffets, or never-ending pasta bowls. Today's food—and I use that term loosely—bears little resemblance to what Americans were fueling their bodies with just twenty-five years ago. More than any other time in our history, we are consuming much more of the calorically dense foods that promote weight gain. That's "energy in." What about "energy out"? I suspect you already know the answer.

How We Work and Live: Sitting Down

In 2011, Dr. Tim Church, professor of preventative medicine at Pennington Biomedical Research Center at Louisiana State University, and his colleagues published an article in *PLoS ONE*. Entitled "Trends over Five Decades in U.S. Occupation-related Physical Activity and Their Associations with Obesity," the article compared how Americans work today versus how we worked in 1960. Using data from the U.S. Bureau of Labor Statistics, researchers determined that in 1960, every five out of ten Americans had a job that required some sort of caloric expenditure (i.e., manual labor). Today, however, that is down to only two out of ten. Partly due to advances in technology in the workplace, many Americans have become what are known as thought workers; we sit all day in front of screens, typing on keyboards, and talking on phones. Compared to 1960, the average man now burns 140 fewer calories per day at work and the average woman, 120 fewer calories.

If you take these trends and lay them over the increase in U.S. obesity rates over the past fifty years, you'll see an amazing correlation. It's no wonder Americans are getting bigger and less fit by the day. Everyone knows the *benefits* of physical activity, but there is growing evidence that a *lack of activity* is quite damaging as well. A study published in the March 26, 2012, issue of the *Archives of Internal Medicine* found that thirty minutes of physical activity a day is "as protective an exposure as ten hours of sitting is a harmful one" (see chapter 6, "Is Sitting the New Smoking?"). The truth is, we have pretty much engineered physical activity *out* of our lives. We have drive-thru banks, restaurants, liquor stores, churches, and wedding chapels—even drive-thru petting zoos. We use remote controls to change the channel, turn on and off the lights, open and close the garage door, and adjust the thermostat. For younger readers: You might not believe it, but years ago, if you wanted to open a car window, you had to turn something called *a handle*. It took about two or three seconds and burned a few calories.

I'm fascinated by a physical-activity study of an Amish population in Ontario, Canada, that was published in a 2004 issue of *Medicine and Science in Sports and Exercise*. The ninety-eight men and women examined exist pretty much as their ancestors lived 150 years ago. They do not drive cars or use electrical appliances. Labor-intensive farming is still the preferred occupation. Before the study, using body mass index (BMI) calculations, researchers found that none of the men and only 9 percent of the women were obese. (Compare that with the current obesity rate of almost 40 percent.) Study participants wore pedometers for a week to track their physical activity. According to data from Katrine Tudor-Locke and John M. Schuna Jr. (published in a 2012 issue of *Research in Exercise Epidemiology*), the average American takes between 5,800 and 7,500 steps a day (there are approximately two thousand steps in a mile), with men averaging more steps than women. In the Amish population studied, however, researchers found that the men averaged more than 18,000 steps per day and the women more than 14,000! They rarely sat during the day, other than for breakfast, lunch, and dinner.

Improving Fitness Offers Benefits Both above the Neck and below the Belt.

As I've mentioned, I believe it's human nature to want to feel and look good. Feeling good is not just about reducing or eliminating *physical* aches and pains, however; it's also about reducing *mental* aches and pains. We all know that life is not linear; it's filled with a series of highs and lows, starts and stops, and often unpredictable speed bumps and even brick walls. It's easy to navigate the peaks. How we handle the valleys is the real challenge. Millions of Americans suffer from some degree of depression, at least occasionally. As it turns out, exercise can help with that.

Large, well-designed clinical studies have shown that exercise not only helps to treat depression but can also help *prevent* depression. A 2016 study of more than 1.1 million adult men and women published in *Preventive Medicine* showed that the link between fitness and depression was significant. Using objective data rather than self-reported measures, the researchers found that those with the lowest fitness levels were 75 percent more likely to have been diagnosed with depression compared against those with the greatest fitness levels. Another big study, this one published in the *Journal of Psychiatric Research* (2016), examined individuals who had been diagnosed with clinical depression to see if exercise might be used as a treatment for depression. The answer is yes, as the authors reported that exercise has a "large and significant effect" against depression. Blood studies may help explain why. Regular exercise significantly reduces inflammation and increases levels of hormones and other biochemicals that are believed to contribute to brain health (as reported in a 2016 issue of *Neuroscience and Biobehavioral Reviews*).

And if you're looking for additional reasons to improve your fitness, there is strong evidence linking fitness levels to enhanced sexual performance and satisfaction, for both men and women. About half of men ages forty to seventy experience some degree of erectile dysfunction (which helps explains all those commercials on TV). Female sexual dysfunction can occur at any age, but the likelihood tends to increase as women grow older, particularly after menopause. The great news is that regular exercise, both aerobic and anaerobic, improves sexual function for both men and women. Specifically, improving your fitness positively affects the endothelium, the inner lining of blood vessels, which helps blood flow more smoothly.

A study published in the *Archives of Sexual Behavior* (1990) showed that men who exercised regularly (sixty minutes a day, three to five days a week, with a sustained peak intensity of 75–80 percent) developed "significantly greater sexual enhancement" (i.e., frequency of various intimate activities, reliability of adequate functioning during sex, and percentage of satisfying orgasms). For ladies, multiple studies, including one published in the *Journal of Sexual Medicine* (2008), found that intense, short-duration exercise (twenty minutes, with a target heart rate of 70 percent) significantly enhances the physiological sexual arousal of women (i.e., genital arousal). It makes sense that when someone loses weight and improves muscle tone, he or she becomes more confident when naked. Confidence is a big part of a healthy sex life, so if you want more boom-boom in the bedroom, be sure to take your dog for a walk . . . even if you don't have a dog!

Taking Responsibility for Your Health

As Americans, many of us have "outsourced" the way we eat, work, and live. It's a much different world than the one our parents and grandparents grew up in, as we've already discussed. The deck is stacked, and today's obesogenic environment isn't very healthy! When you connect all these dots, it may sound as if I'm being rather fatalistic, but nothing could be further from the truth. I know from both personal and professional experience that embracing healthy behaviors can make an *enormous* difference in your life; however, it's going to take a personal commitment and a plan.

There are more than seven and a half billion people in the world, and not one of them can eat for you or move for you. Your health doesn't depend on the government, your doctor, your employer, or your significant other. It is *your* responsibility! Invest in yourself. If you need to improve your health, then seek council. Read, research, go to lectures. Hire a trainer or visit a dietitian. Improve your understanding of what it takes to be healthy, then strategically figure out how to embrace a lifestyle that will result in more energy, better sleep, an enhanced sex life, improved risk factors, less depression, higher self-esteem, and more options as you age! This book is chock-full of ideas to put you on a path toward healthy living.

Poor health limits your opportunities. There's a big difference between living and being alive. Every aspect of your life is enhanced when your health improves, so take charge and get started. One month from now, you will either be healthier or less healthy than you are today. In which direction are you headed? To quote rock legends Led Zeppelin:

"Yes, there are two paths you can go by, but in the long run / There's still time to change the road you're on."
("Stairway to Heaven")

"Do not fear failure, fear average."

3.

Get to Goal:
You Are What Your Risk Factors Say You Are

Fans of pro football will recognize this quotation from Bill Parcells, two-time Super Bowl champion coach of the New York Giants: "You are what your record says you are." Basically, if you have a four-and-twelve record, you have a bad football team! You can't sugarcoat it; the record speaks for itself. In health, there is a similar saying: You are what your risk factors say you are. Technically, a risk factor is a variable associated with an increased risk of disease or infection. There is an inverse relationship between risk factors and health: The fewer risk factors you have, the better health you enjoy. Conversely, the more risk factors you have, the greater the likelihood you currently are (or will be) in poor health.

Some risk factors, you can't change. They are nonmodifiable and include your age, gender, and family history (e.g., if your dad and grandfather died of heart disease before they were fifty). You have control over other risk factors, however. These include your fitness level, weight, alcohol consumption, tobacco use, and blood pressure, as well as your cholesterol, glucose, vitamin D levels, and so on (for more on optimal vitamin D levels, see chapter 26, "What about Supplements?"). You can almost always improve these risk factors by changing your habits and lifestyle. The body is beautifully designed to do what you ask it to do. If you treat yourself well more times than not, the body will respond in an amazing manner. On the contrary, if you treat yourself poorly (by smoking, not exercising, eating large amounts of crummy food, not getting enough sleep, or abusing alcohol), then your health will suffer.

Remember, you are *not* standing still in terms of your health. Either you are in decline or you are improving. Please don't think that just because you are getting older, your health automatically needs to suffer. At just about any stage of life, if you put your mind (and body) to it, you can reverse or at least slow a negative slide. I encourage you to get a handle on your risk factors. The first step is to get a very thorough comprehensive medical exam (i.e., a physical). This can be done by a good general-practice doctor—or if you're so inclined, you can get what's called an executive physical at a facility like the Mayo Clinic (campuses are in Minnesota, Arizona, and Florida), Cleveland Clinic (Ohio), Cooper Clinic (Dallas), or Johns Hopkins (Maryland). Although the definition of an executive physical varies greatly, it often includes expanded blood work to measure emerging coronary risk factors such as C-reactive protein and IL-6 (both measures of systemic inflammation) and LDL-cholesterol particle size, a maximal stress test (even for asymptomatic patients), and screening using ultrafast CT imagery to assess coronary calcification (the amount of plaque in the arteries of the heart).

There is great debate in the medical community about whether these tests should even be considered in healthy, asymptomatic individuals because of what is known as "number needed to treat." In other words, you might have to test 1,000 individuals, at considerable expense, to save just one life. Many health economists consider that a waste of money, which is true—unless, of course, you happen to be that one in 1,000. Although insurance usually does not cover these more extensive evaluations, the exams are excellent at providing a terrific baseline. With the information provided by them, you and your doctor can develop a game plan for the future.

If you have areas of risk, you should, as doctors love to say, get to goal. It's always best to try to achieve your goals through lifestyle modification first, but if that doesn't work, don't rule out medications. For example, high blood pressure can often be lowered by changing your diet and losing weight;

however, some people do *everything possible* in terms of healthy habits yet still have issues. If you fall into this category, don't pretend that the problem is going to go away just because you ignore it. Have an open and honest conversation with your doctor about this.

As President John Kennedy said, "The time to repair the roof is when the sun is shining." Please don't wait until you have symptoms—that may be too late! The most common symptom of heart disease is not chest pain, shortness of breath, or nausea—it's *death*! As published in a 2010 issue of the *American Journal of Clinical Nutrition*, 55 percent of men and 68 percent of women who die of sudden cardiac death have never been diagnosed with heart disease ("Plasma and Dietary Magnesium and Risk of Sudden Cardiac Death in Women, by Stephanie E. Chiuve et al.). Don't let yourself become a statistic. Know your risk factors, and get to goal!

Your Annual Physical

Most physicians love data, and a comprehensive blood test is the perfect way to start gathering data. Having accurate measurements help doctors determine if you have any immediate areas of concern. This blood work should include your total cholesterol, HDL cholesterol, LDL cholesterol, triglycerides, blood glucose, vitamin D, C-reactive protein, and, ideally, HS-Omega-3 Index. Your exam should also include a check of your blood pressure, height and weight (to determine body mass index, BMI), and waist circumference. As of 2014, 54 percent of American adults have excess belly fat, which is associated with a much greater risk of such dangerous conditions as heart disease, stroke, certain cancers, and maybe even Alzheimer's disease. ("Excess" is defined as a waist circumference greater than forty inches for a man and thirty-five inches for a woman.)

As we get older, our key risk factors often change dramatically despite any major change in lifestyle—that is, weight, diet, or activity level. That's why it makes sense for people over the age of forty to get physicals at least every two years. Don't be guilty of the "I feel fine" syndrome (something especially prevalent among men, but women can fall prey to this as well). *Feeling* fine doesn't necessarily mean you *are* fine.

Make sure your physical includes age- and gender-specific preventive screens, such as, for men, a prostate exam, as well as a PSA (prostate specific antigen) test. Best practices for women include a mammogram and a Pap smear. For both men and women, please remember the importance of a colonoscopy. Don't set yourself up for long-term health risks by trying to protect yourself from short-term embarrassment!

Probably the most important part of your annual physical is known by physicians as the consult. This is your chance to sit one-on-one with your doctor and discuss the results. In today's health-care environment, time has become a precious commodity for most doctors, meaning your consult may be conducted by a physician's assistant or a nurse practitioner. That's not a problem, as long as he or she is thorough, clear, and willing to listen. If you are not medically trained yourself, you may want to take notes or use your phone to record the consult. That way, you can go back later and pick up any comments or suggestions you may have missed. As a patient, you are the customer, so make sure you get all of your questions answered. Better yet, before the consult, take a few minutes to write down a list of any questions you might have, and be sure to ask them—that way, you'll be sure you've covered everything.

Finding a Good Doctor

Doctors have the greatest influence on getting us to change our behaviors. Ideally, find a doctor or healthcare professional who has the time and training to talk to you about such topics as nutrition and exercise. I'm a huge advocate of using healthy lifestyle choices to correct adverse risk factors whenever possible. Be sure to talk to your doctor about all the options you might have before he or she pulls out the prescription pad.

Not all doctors are created equal. I'm often asked how to find a good one. There's no magic formula, but a great place to start is by asking friends, neighbors, or colleagues for their recommendations. When it comes to your health, don't compromise. Once you find a doctor you're comfortable with, let him or her help you manage your risk factors, but ultimately your health is your responsibility, not your doctor's.

> "If you do not change direction,
> you may end up where you are heading."
> - Lao Tzu

"If you've got your health, you're a zillionaire!"
- Dick Vitale

4.

Beware the Escalator: From Prediabetes to Diabetes

When I was very young, around three or four, my mother would take my hand and lift me into the air as we approached an escalator. I looked at it as a game, but she made the consequences very clear: If you weren't paying attention, you could get a shoelace caught in the sharp grates and possibly lose a foot or a leg. Little did I know how prophetic my mom was. Indeed, escalators can be incredibly dangerous.

My colleague Den Bishop, a very smart dude, has a gift for simplifying complex topics. Take, for instance, his metaphor illustrating the progression from being healthy to developing diabetes. That doesn't happen overnight. It's all about the escalator. Imagine a department store. On the first floor is the Healthy Department. People who hang out here have glucose levels of 100 mg/dL (milligrams per deciliter) or below. On the second floor of the department store is the Diabetes Department. To be on this level, your glucose level must be 126 mg/dL or higher. Connecting the first and second floors is an escalator. (Have you ever noticed that most department stores don't have stairs?) As you have probably already guessed, the folks on the escalator have glucose levels between 100 to 125 mg/dL.

Now comes the important question: If you find yourself on an escalator, what must you do to get to the next floor? The answer is . . . nothing. Nothing at all. The power and momentum of the escalator will simply drop you off on the next level—in this case, the Diabetes Department. Having a blood glucose level between 100 and 125 means you are prediabetic. If you don't start exercising and lose some weight when you are in the prediabetic phase, it's not a matter of *if* you will develop diabetes but a matter of *when*. If you do nothing, the escalator will simply carry you to the Diabetes Department, where you will be assigned a personal shopper, otherwise known as a case management nurse or critical care nurse.

As of 2012, about 50 percent of American adults are in the Healthy Department, at least when it comes to diabetic risk. A little over 12 percent are already diabetic. But here's what's scary: According to the American Diabetes Association, 37 percent of adults are on the diabetes escalator, and nine out of ten of them don't know even know it. The latest data indicate that in the United States, 49.3 percent of adults are either diabetic or prediabetic. Each and every day, more than 4,600 individuals step off the escalator and onto a floor where, most likely, their lives will never be the same.

The trend is not getting better; in fact, it's getting worse. The Centers for Disease Control and Prevention announced in 2014 that 40 percent of Americans born between 2000 and 2011 will develop type 2 diabetes in their lifetimes. This is double the risk of those born just a decade earlier. The numbers are even more ominous for people of color: More than half of all Hispanics and of non-Hispanic black women born between 2000 and 2011 will develop diabetes in their lifetimes. For black men, the lifetime risk is 45 percent. Think about these predictions. More than 100 million Americans will have a disease that is entirely avoidable. For the most part, type 2 diabetes is a human-made disease, meaning that it is a lifestyle disease and the result of people making unhealthy choices. (Type 1 diabetes is primarily genetic.) The financial cost will be enormous, to be sure, but what about the societal cost? The impact on quality of life? With diabetes, the risks of heart attack and stroke increase exponentially. The painful condition known as peripheral neuropathy becomes a daily companion. Kidney failure is common. Fatty liver disease kicks in. Eventually, poor circulation can lead to blindness and amputation.

I do quite a bit of speaking around the country to various groups. When I share these statistics, I'm fascinated by some of the responses. Sometimes I hear gasps or such comments as "Oh my goodness!" or "I had no idea!" Business owners and corporate leaders are realizing that managing healthcare means more than just switching insurance carriers, increasing deductibles, or implementing other forms of cost shifting (pushing the increases to the employees). Others don't seem too bothered by the dire statistics, however. Perhaps they are mistakenly thinking, *Hey, if I'm in the Healthy Department, then it's not my problem.* Nothing could be further from the truth, unfortunately. Each one of us will pay the price for the diabetes epidemic. Young and old, rich and poor, healthy and unhealthy, everyone will be forced to share in the cost. We have to pay attention to the escalator!

"We should all be concerned with the future,
because we're going to spend the rest of our lives there."
– Charles F. Kettering

"If we did all the things we are capable of,
we would literally astound ourselves."
– Thomas Edison

5.

Indicators of Health and Risk:
BMI and Body Fat Percentage

Many of us, especially men, like to keep score. Wanting to know how we compare to others is a fairly common human trait. Quite often, I am asked about the body mass index, or BMI, and whether it's something to worry about. The answer is yes . . . and no. BMI is simply a height-weight ratio. The concept was invented by the insurance industry to easily and cost-effectively assess an individual's health and risk of disease. For adults, the easiest way to calculate BMI is simply to Google "BMI." The Internet has dozens of free BMI calculators. Fill in your height and weight, hit Enter, and you'll see where you stand.

If you are old-school and want to calculate your BMI by hand, take your weight in pounds and multiply by 703. Then, divide that result by your height in inches. Now, divide that number a second time by your height in inches (The formula is the same for both men and women.) A BMI of 18.5–24.9 defines a "normal weight." A BMI between 25 and 29.9 is considered overweight, and a BMI of 30 or more is considered obese. A rough ballpark estimation of obesity is thirty or more pounds overweight. "Morbid obesity" (Class III) is defined as a BMI of 40 or greater and is roughly the equivalent of being at least one hundred pounds overweight. These definitions are very objective. BMI is simply a definition based on a mathematical calculation. Often, people become offended when a doctor or health professional tells them they fall into the overweight or obese categories. It's nothing personal, just a fact based on the definitions and the BMI formula. (The BMI calculations for children and teens are different. They are available online at www.cdc.gov/healthyweight/assessing/bmi/childrens_bmi/about_childrens_bmi.html.)

One caveat about BMI: If you are naturally lean and athletic or heavily muscled (think Mike Tyson in his prime, before he started biting ears), your BMI is not of much value. For example, when Tyson was at his peak as a boxer, he was 5'10" and weighed 223 pounds. That would give him a BMI of 33.4, well into the range for obesity. Obviously, Tyson was more ripped than obese. If you are very lean—not "skinny," but lean—there's no need to pay much attention to your BMI.

My advice? Be aware of your BMI but don't completely obsess over it; because many Americans are not lifting weights or are not naturally muscled, BMI should be considered just one helpful piece of data in determining your overall health. But know that this number can definitely affect your life insurance rates, and depending on where you work, it might also affect what you pay for health insurance.

Predicting Health Risks

Some argue that BMI is not a great indicator of health risks because the number does not account for body shape, fat mass, and lean mass; however, a study published in the November 2012 issue of *Obesity Research & Clinical Practice* indicates otherwise. Researchers compared BMI, body fat percentage, waist circumference, and waist-to-height ratio for more than 12,000 men and women. They calculated how well each measure predicted elements of metabolic syndrome, including high blood pressure, elevated fasting glucose, reduced HDL ("good") cholesterol, and raised LDL ("bad") cholesterol. (Metabolic syndrome, or MetS, increases the risk of heart disease, stroke and Type 2 diabetes.)

Although some of the measurements were slightly better at predicting particular risks, none were consistently better than BMI at predicting all of these risk factors. Thus, you should not ignore your BMI, even if you don't agree with the definition. As Scottish philosopher David Hume once quipped, "A wise man proportions his belief to the evidence."

I have another simple and highly effective method for figuring out if you are height-weight appropriate. Go into the bathroom. Shut and lock the door. Disrobe. Now stand in front of the mirror and jump up and down. Some body parts are designed to move, and some are not. You will know whether you might benefit from dropping a few pounds after doing this (although I suspect you probably already know). A much more scientific method of assessing your particular body composition is to determine your body fat percentage. This is a great piece of data but is tougher to calculate than BMI is. Your total body weight comprises organs (heart, liver, kidneys, and so on), bones, water, fat, and muscle. The real variables are fat and muscle. The greater the amount of fat you carry as a percentage of total weight, especially visceral (or belly) fat, the greater the likelihood that your health will be negatively affected. Conversely, the more lean muscle you have as a percentage of total weight, the better.

You can determine your body fat percentage a number of ways. The most accurate is the DEXA (dual-energy X-ray absorptiometry) scan, which many women are familiar with because that's also the best way to measure bone density. Other methods include hydrostatic (underwater) weighing, skin calipers (skin fold), and bioelectrical impedance analysis (bioimpedance, or BIA) using special scales. There are plusses and minuses to all of these methods, including accuracy, availability, simplicity, and cost.

If you get your body fat percentage measured using skin calipers, make sure that whoever conducts the test has been properly certified; otherwise, your results might not be reliable. If you use a body fat scale (a BIA scale), make sure to measure yourself at the same time every day, because your hydration level will affect the result. Most people do it first thing in the morning right after voiding (a technical way of saying "urinating"). Although these scales are not considered the gold standard in terms of accuracy, they are helpful in identifying trends, especially if you are beginning to lift weights. Many times, when people start to weight train while also dieting, they add lean muscle and lose body fat. Their weight and BMI often don't change much, which can be frustrating, but in reality, their body composition is moving in a positive direction. (Tanita and Omron are two reliable brands of BIA scales. Prices start at about forty dollars.)

Unlike BMI, categories of body fat percentage are different for men and women. Men carry more muscle (both in percentage and in total muscle) than do women and therefore generally are leaner. Here are the categories for body fat percentage from the American College of Sports Medicine, based on data from the Cooper Institute in Dallas:

ACSM Body Composition (% Body Fat) For Men and Women

Male

Percentile	Fitness Category	20-29	AGE 30-39	40-49	50-59	60+
90	Well Above Average	7.1-11.7	11.3-15.8	13.6-18	15.3-19.7	15.3-20.7
70	Above Average	11.8-15.8	15.9-18.9	18.1-21	19.8-22.6	20.8-23.4
50	Average	15.9-19.4	19-22.2	21.1-24	22.7-25.6	23.5-26.6
30	Below Average	19.5-25.8	22.3-27.2	24.1-28.8	25.7-30.2	26.7-31.1
10	Well Below Average	25.9	27.3	28.9	30.3	31.2

Female

Percentile	Fitness Category	20-29	AGE 30-39	40-49	50-59	60+
90	Well Above Average	14.5-18.9	15.5-19.9	18.5-23.4	21.6-26.5	21.1-27.4
70	Above Average	19-22	20-23	23.5-26.3	26.6-30	27.5-30.8
50	Average	22.1-25.3	23.1-26.9	26.4-30	30.1-33.4	30.9-34.2
30	Below Average	25.4-32	27-32.7	30.1-34.9	33.5-37.8	34.3-39.2
10	Well Below Average	32.1	32.8	35	37.9	39.3

*Data provided by the Institute for Aerobics Research, Dallas, TX (1994). Study population for the data set was predominately White and college educated.

Taken from ACSM'S Health-Related Physical Fitness Assessment Manual, 2ndEd. 2008. pg 59.

Reprinted with permission of ACSM/Wolters Kluwer Health

As men and women age, we lose muscle mass—a condition known as sarcopenia, or muscle wasting. That means our body fat percentage generally goes up with age. The best way to prevent that, or at least to slow the progression, is to engage in regular strength-training exercises. This could look different depending on your likes and dislikes, so choose what appeals to you: lifting free weights, using weight machines, practicing yoga, Pilates, working with kettlebells, doing plyometric exercises (also called "jump training"), etc. I'm a big fan of variety, which helps to continually challenge the body and keep you mentally fresh.

Listen to the Experts

I advocate relying on experts, such as personal trainers, to assist you in developing an effective strength-training program. Not all personal trainers are created equal, so find one who is experienced and credentialed and who listens to what your goals and objectives are. Trainers can be a great source of motivation. You certainly don't need a trainer for every workout, but fine-tuning your routine fairly regularly (every two to three months) makes sense. Mixing it up will help you improve your results.

Everyone, both men and women, should focus on achieving and maintaining a healthy body fat percentage. Women, don't be intimidated by strength training! You'll be amazed at how it can help shape your body. It also can help eliminate any jiggle you might have when performing the "parade wave" (think the Queen of England). Proper weight training (along with regular doses of calcium and vitamin D) can dramatically improve bone density, which will significantly reduce the risk of osteopenia and osteoporosis. Statistically, one out of every two women will eventually develop osteoporosis (and one out of every five or six men). Don't let that be you! If you've already been diagnosed with either of those conditions or think you might be at risk, be sure to get clearance from your doctor before starting a weight-lifting program.

The bottom line: BMI is something to pay attention to, but it's not the only health factor to consider. *How* you weigh (your body composition) is much more important than *what* you weigh (the number on the scale). Don't define yourself, or your health, by your weight; it's *a* factor but certainly not the *only* factor.

> "I can't believe that God put us on this earth to be ordinary."
> – Lou Holtz

"What saves a man is to take a step.
Then another step.
It is always the same step, but you have to take it."
– Antoine de Saint-Exupery

6.

Is Sitting the New Smoking?

The enormous benefits of exercise have been well documented in hundreds of scientific publications. There can't be many Americans who don't know that exercise does a body good. But now we're learning something new, and it's pretty frightening: Sitting is detrimental to your health—especially sitting for long periods of time. While physical activity (i.e., exercise) is beneficial, it appears that physical *inactivity* is very dangerous.

Let's take a look at the emerging data. An article by Genevieve N. Healy et al. ("Breaks in Sedentary Time: Beneficial Associations with Metabolic Risk") published in the April 2008 issue of *Diabetes Care* reported that frequent breaks in sedentary activity may explain lower health risk related to waist circumference, BMI, triglyceride levels, and two-hour plasma glucose levels. These risk factors, along with triglyceride and HDL levels, define metabolic syndrome (as mentioned in Chapter 5).

A study published in a 2012 issue of *Archives of Internal Medicine* ("Sitting Time and All-Cause Mortality Risk in 222,497 Australian Adults," by Hidde P. van der Ploeg et al.) concluded that thirty minutes of physical activity is as protective an exposure as ten hours of sitting is a harmful one. Also in 2012, the *British Journal of Sports Medicine* indicated that one hour of sitting is the equivalent of smoking two cigarettes. Holy smokes! Think about that—especially if you have a desk job that pays you to sit and stare at a screen, type on a keyboard, and talk on the phone all day. According to Professor David W. Dunston, a researcher associated with the Australian Obesity, Diabetes, and Lifestyle Study, the most striking feature of prolonged sitting is the absence of skeletal muscle contractions, particularly in the large muscles of the legs (quads, hamstrings, and calf muscles).

This should be rather alarming, especially in light of Dr. Tim Church's 2011 study that was discussed in chapter 2, which notes that today, only one in five US workers is physically active on the job. Most all of us are thought workers, compensated for our brains, not for our bodies. We get paid to sit, think, and move information around electronically!

This new body of evidence is also concerning for those who are retired. A 2014 article published in the *Journal of Physical Activity and Health* found that "for those sixty and older, every additional hour per day of sitting is linked to a 50 percent greater risk of being disabled . . . regardless of the amount of moderate physical activity you get." Wow! Even if you exercise thirty or sixty minutes a day, prolonged "couch potato" behavior will still dramatically increase your risk of becoming disabled.

What can be done? Simple: Stand up! Regularly. The simple act of getting out of your chair every thirty to sixty minutes has tremendous benefit. All the better if you're willing to do some toe-raisers, desk push-ups, or chair squats. A short walk around the office works wonders, as well. It doesn't have to be much or be long; just a couple of minutes every hour or so is all it takes. Using the alarm on your smartphone can serve as a reminder (i.e., a trigger). Add in a simple incentive or two, some social engagement, and you would be amazed how easy it is to change your deskbound behavior. Health is mostly a function of habits. Unhealthy habits, like prolonged bouts of sitting, over time are extremely damaging. Pay attention to the science, and intentionally develop ways to put your body in a position to function at its peak for years to come. .

"Yes, exercise is the catalyst. That's what makes everything happen: your digestion, your elimination, your sex life, your skin, hair, everything about you depends on circulation. And how do you increase circulation?"
– Jack LaLanne

"Without ambition, one starts nothing.
Without work, one finishes nothing.
The prize will not be sent to you.
You have to win in."
– Ralph Waldo Emerson

7.

Make the Investment and Improve Your Odds

I don't have an ounce of data to support what I'm about to share, but here it is: An appreciation of the future might significantly improve your odds of living a longer, more fulfilling life. It's just a theory, something for you to think about.

Embracing healthy habits can not only extend your life by six to nine years but also help push back the onset of disability by between thirteen and twenty years. My parents spent their final years physically and psychologically challenged, so I am driven to not let that happen to me. From my perspective, it makes total sense to eat right, exercise regularly, avoid smoking, brush and floss my teeth, get plenty of sleep, moderate my alcohol intake, manage stress, get an annual physical, and take the right supplements (for more on my top three recommended supplements, see Chapter 26). Why wouldn't everyone do that? For me, the research is impossible to argue with. Just do the right things and you will, at least statistically, dramatically improve your odds of living a long and full life.

Even though that concept is easy to understand, it's not necessarily enough to motivate permanent behavior change. The reason, I believe, is that the majority of benefits from a healthy lifestyle happen down the road, not today or tomorrow. Today's investment doesn't show a return until, sometimes, much later. Most of us tend to think more about *now* than the future. Most of us don't want to think about what our lives will be like when we're older. We think anything bad or negative will happen to someone else, not us.

Why would people continue to smoke when they know it dramatically increases their odds of developing lung cancer and heart disease? I believe most people simply aren't wired to think that far out.

Dr. Elliott Jacques's Time Span

Dr. Elliott Jacques was a fascinating man. Born in Canada, he received an MD from Johns Hopkins and a PhD from Harvard. He spent his entire career studying how to build the most efficient teams within business organizations. He wrote twenty books, but much of his research boiled down to what he defined as "time span," or "the length of time a person can work into the future, without direction, using discretionary judgment, to achieve a specific goal" (*Time Span Handbook*, 1964).

Let me explain this a bit further. Basically, if you give someone a job or task to accomplish, how far into the future can you set a deadline for him or her to successfully get the job done? Dr. Jacques believed that an individual's time span is innate and that it is independent of IQ. He broke time span into stratums. People who are in Strata I can work about three months into the future. They generally don't save much money, participate in a 401(k) plan, or think a great deal about down the road. They think mostly about what they plan to do that night or weekend. In a normal corporate environment, these people generally are paid hourly and work on the front lines. Strata I individuals are all about production and often work as technicians, equipment operators, or clerks, or in data entry. Dr. Jacques believed that about 40 percent of people are in Strata I.

Strata II individuals, another 40 percent of adults, can work about one year into the future. They can do some scheduling and can usually be relied on to follow a regular maintenance schedule. In a large company, Strata II folks often work as supervisors, coordinators, project managers, engineers, and line managers. These are the individuals who make sure production happens. If the goal or project has a deadline of more than a year, however, Strata II folks will often not be able to accomplish the task. It will be frustrating for them and also for those they report to (and for those who report to them).

As you go up the time-span ladder, the populations get smaller and smaller. Strata III individuals, who make up about 7 percent of the general population, can see two years out. They are the ones who create the production systems and work as unit managers, plant managers, and operations managers.

According to Dr. Jacques, only 1 percent of the population falls into the Strata IV category. With this group, the vision is between two and five years and includes general managers, chief operations officers, and chief financial officers.

Obviously, the category of Strata V is not large at all: 0.07 percent of those ages twenty-one to fifty, only seven in every ten thousand people! These are the CEOs or, in a really large company, the business unit presidents. Their time span is more than five years.

Short-Term Pleasure versus Long-Term Benefit

What does any of this have to do with health and wellness? Dr. Jacques felt that at any given time, 10 percent of the population would be either unemployed or unemployable. If you add that 10 percent to individuals in the Strata I and Strata II categories, that means 90 percent of adults aren't wired to think more than about a year into the future. Even though the majority of Americans might understand the concept of living exceptionally, it really isn't going to be motivating enough for them to go for a walk rather than sit and binge-watch their favorite TV show. Theoretically, for many people, opting for steamed veggies rather than french fries is not going to happen because the fries taste so amazingly good *right now* and the risk of cardiovascular disease or diabetes is something that *might* happen way down the road.

Again, I don't have a shred of evidence to support this idea, but it might explain why so many Americans succumb to choices that result in short-term pleasure rather than long-term benefit. When you start an exercise or nutrition program, it can sometimes be months before you see or feel the results of all your hard work. With the advances in today's technology, we've come to appreciate instant gratification; "now" is much more fun than "later." If you factor in all of the obesogenic environmental influences such as fast food (which is cheap, convenient, and engineered to manipulate us into becoming addicted) and a sedentary lifestyle, is it any wonder that nearly 40 percent of Americans are now obese?

The experts at VitalSmarts, a leadership consulting firm, speak of the importance of identifying your "default future." In essence, if you continue living as you are now, what will your life look like in ten, twenty, thirty, even fifty years? Will you be able to do the things you enjoy today? As mentioned earlier, a healthy lifestyle will help you push back the onset of disability by up to twenty years. That's an amazing statistic, but to make that happen, you need to establish—and practice—good habits today (and tomorrow). Is that possible? Absolutely! An appreciation of the future might significantly improve your odds!

> "You will never change your life
> until you change something you do daily."
> – Mike Murdoch

> "Success is the sum of small efforts
> repeated day in and day out."
> – Robert Collier

8.

The Dose Counts: Embracing Moderation

Whenever someone tells me he or she takes a supplement, say omega-3 or vitamin D, I ask, "How much?" More times than not, the response is something like "one tablet" or "two pills." When I ask how much is in each dose, I usually get a blank stare.

I get it. Unless you spend a great deal of time studying this type of stuff, it can be confusing. Some consumers don't know the difference between a milligram, a microgram, and a telegram, let alone an international unit.

What you *need* to know is that the dose counts. Almost everything has a beneficial range: Too little won't make any difference, and too much can cause problems. You need to shoot for the sweet spot, known in scientific terms as the therapeutic window. When you think about it, everything has an appropriate dose: minutes of exercise, hours of sleep, squirts of condiments, teaspoons of sugar in your coffee, even the amount of water you drink daily. If you're really thirsty, a thimbleful of water certainly won't quench your thirst, but drinking a five-gallon jug would be dangerous. Somewhere in between is the proper amount, or dose, that will satisfy your needs and provide benefit.

Moderation is key! Making too many changes too soon will be harder to sustain over the long term. Throughout this book are recommendations for all sorts of things. Shoot for the range (or minimum dose) that you need to accomplish your personal goals, whatever they may be. These recommendations are important. It's not just the ingredient or the activity that counts, it's also the appropriate dose!

> "A small daily task, if it be really daily,
> will beat the labours of a spasmodic Hercules."
> – Anthony Trollope

PART 2

Embracing Healthy Behaviors

"Our body is a machine for living.
It is organized for that, it is its nature."
– Leo Tolstoy

9.

Cut the Crap: Quality Matters

I was born in 1957, which means I'm old enough to remember a lot of fad diets. The first diet I consciously became aware of was the grapefruit diet. This one actually started in the 1930s, but it got hot again in the 1970s. "Just eat half of a grapefruit with every meal for ten to twelve days, and the pounds will melt away!" This plan made no sense to me, probably because I've never been a fan of grapefruit.

There have been plenty of other fad diets over the years: the coffee diet; the cabbage soup diet; the lemonade, chocolate, and acai berry diets. It seems that every couple of years, we hear about the latest and greatest fast and simple solution to shed pounds effortlessly, always without exercise. Some seem *really* out there, like the apple cider vinegar diet. Then there are the HCG (human chorionic gonadotropin), blood type, body ecology, flavor point, hot Latin, warrior, martini, and hallelujah diets. And don't forget Atkins and South Beach. The list goes on and on and on, each espousing the secret to weight loss.

Over the past decade or so, Americans have been subjected to a whole new round of "solutions"—not diets, per se, but "lifestyle" ways of eating: low-carb, paleo, gluten-free (Note: I am not referring here to those who must eat a gluten-free diet because they have celiac disease—a very real condition and most definitely not a fad!), ketogenic, Whole30, vegan, eco-Atkins, low-glycemic index, intermittent fasting, Portfolio vegetarian, and so on.

Of interest from a public health perspective, not one of these diets has made, as my dad used to say, a hill of beans' difference. In fact, as a nation, Americans are bigger and less healthy than we've ever been. Ever! In 1962, 13 percent of American adults were obese. As of 2017, 39.8 percent of American adults are obese—and, as you know, we're growing. (As discussed in Chapter 5, a BMI of 30 or greater equates to about thirty pounds overweight, and a BMI of 40 or greater—considered class III, or morbid, obesity—is about one hundred pounds overweight.) All this despite the multibillion dollar diet industry! What does this tell us? Simply stated: Diets don't work! I'm not planning to write a diet book, but if I ever did, I have the title ready to go: *The Cut-the-Crap Diet!* (pardon my French). Food is the body's fuel. There's a lot more to eating than consuming calories. Yes, the *quantity* is certainly a factor to consider, but I believe that *quality* is of even greater importance.

Look around. What are people consuming? Obviously, there is tremendous variance, but overall, many Americans are eating "food" that offers little nutritional value. It's cheap, convenient, and craveable, thanks to lab-perfected levels of salt-fat-sugar ratios. But we were not designed to eat this way. That isn't the type of fuel that that will allow our bodies to thrive.

Entire books have been written about the deplorable state of food options in the United States, reporting pretty disturbing realities. I highly suggest reading *Salt Sugar Fat: How the Food Giants Hooked Us,* by Michael Moss; *The Omnivore's Dilemma: A Natural History of Four Meals,* by Michael Pollan; *Fast Food Nation: The Dark Side of the All-American Meal,* by Eric Schlosser; and *The End of Overeating: Taking Control of the Insatiable American Appetite,* by David Kessler; and *Disease Proof,* by David Katz. If you prefer movies, watch *Food, Inc.*; *Super Size Me,* and *King Corn. Forks over Knives* is also worth watching, but it clearly has an agenda. I would stay away from the movie version of *Fast Food Nation;* I loved the book, but couldn't watch the movie.

Airport Stories: Cinnabons and Soda

Because I travel a great deal for my work, I spend quite a bit of time in airports. I marvel at what many people are doing to themselves. Not long ago, I spoke in Las Vegas and had a return flight to Dallas early the next morning. While I was waiting at my gate, a young guy, somewhere in his mid-twenties, sat down across from me. He took out his laptop and put on his headphones. This was a large man. My guess would be 6' or 6'1" and at least 320 pounds, maybe more. After getting situated, he reached down and pulled a huge Cinnabon out of a bag, along with a thirty-two-ounce soft drink. Here it was, six-something in the morning, and he was loading close to a thousand calories of crud into his body. According to Cinnabon's website, this guy's breakfast was the pièce de résistance: "It's the roll that made us famous! Warm dough filled with our legendary Makara® Cinnamon, topped with rich cream cheese frosting." This "classic" has 880 calories, with 36 grams of fat (17 of which are saturated), 830 milligrams of sodium (salt), and 59 grams of sugar.

If my neighbor at the gate was eating the Caramel Pecanbon, he was ingesting 1,080 calories, 50 grams of fat (20 of which are saturated), 960 milligrams of sodium, and 76 grams of sugar! If the soft drink was regular (rather than diet), toss on an additional 370 or so calories, 104 grams of sugar, and 120 milligrams of sodium. What nutrition do you get from a breakfast like that? High fructose corn syrup and sodium (salt) with zero fiber, zero protein, and zero vitamin A, vitamin C, calcium, or iron. My friend would need to walk for over an hour and a half (ninety-six minutes) to burn the amount of calories from ingesting just the soft drink, not counting the Cinnabon.

On another recent morning flight from Dallas to Baltimore, I was sitting in the window seat of an exit row. The middle seat was empty, and there was a guy probably in his forties in the aisle seat. When the flight attendant came by taking orders, my row mate ordered a double Bloody Mary and potato chips. (I realize what

I'm about to say sounds extremely judgmental, but I prefer to think of it as merely hyper-observational.) While the double Bloody Mary opens the possibility of all sorts of discussion, I was most intrigued with the chips. They were Boxer Chips, made in Dublin, Ireland. On the brightly colored packaging, the chips were promoted as "savagely salted . . . but not indecently so!" I would beg to differ. I couldn't check my neighbor's chips without fear of reprisal, and I was unable to get the nutritional info from the company's website (they did not return my e-mails), but by my best estimate for the bag is 870 milligrams of sodium, or 38 percent of what is suggested the upper limit we should consume in an entire day (2,300 milligrams).

The topic of salt consumption has been hotly debated in the scientific community. From a basic physiological standpoint, adult men require between 180 and 500 milligrams of sodium per day; 1,500 milligrams is considered the "recommended adequate intake level," and 2,300 milligrams the "tolerable upper intake." The Centers for Disease Control report that the average sodium intake for Americans ages two and up is way higher than that: 3,436 milligrams per day. High sodium intake can increase blood pressure, which is a major risk factor for heart disease and stroke.

We can all find similar examples of poor nutritional choices like these in our communities: in a convenience store, a mall food court (don't get me started on the food options at malls), or a school lunchroom (minus the Bloody Mary, of course). My point is simple. We are losing the battle. The big food companies produce crap that is almost impossible to resist. It's engineered to trigger responses in our brains that drive what food scientists refer to as craveability.

That, by the way, is a tremendous business model. If you could figure out a way to get people to crave your product, wouldn't that be great? Not *like* or *appreciate*, but actually *crave*! You would be rich in a hurry! You can't blame the suppliers—at least not from a business perspective. They get it. They understand that the probability of heart disease, cancer, obesity, and diabetes pales in comparison to the incredible allure of the hot, crunchy-on-the-outside, soft-on-the-inside french fries perfectly salted and dipped in high-fructose corn syrup (aka ketchup) that are calling your name while you're sitting in the line at the drive-thru.

For years, dieticians and health professionals have been chanting," Eat more fruits and vegetables! Five (servings) is fine, but nine is divine, and eleven is heaven!" How's that been working? The results of a ten-year national campaign, Healthy Eating 2010, found that after a decade of public health messaging, only 32.5 percent of Americans eat two servings of fruit and 26.3 percent eat three servings of veggies a day.

Defining "Food"

The experts claim it's easier to start a new habit than to break an existing one. I don't doubt this, but I encourage you to cut the crap! Quit fooling yourself. Be mindful of what you put in your mouth. As Michael Pollan asks, is this food (something your great-grandmother would recognize), or is it a man-made food-like substance (i.e., crap)? Consider whether the food ever had life. Did it grow from the ground, a plant, or a tree? Did it ever have a mother? If so, that's food. Food is not something that was engineered in a lab by "food scientists" who know exactly how to pull levers and tweak dials to make our brains do cartwheels.

In 2014, Yale researchers David Katz and Stephanie Meller, in their article "Can We Say What Diet Is Best for Health?" (published in the *Annual Review of Public Health*), reviewed all of the various diets currently promoted in the United States and came away with a simple recommendation: "A diet of minimally processed foods close to nature, predominantly plants, is decisively associated with health promotion and disease prevention and is consistent with the salient components of seemingly distinct dietary approaches." In other words, there is no single winner when it comes to diets or eating styles, despite what many of the best-selling authors and so-called experts will tell you. It all boils down to Professor Pollan's simple yet brilliant mantra from his *In Defense of Food: An Eater's Manifesto*: "Eat food. Not too much. Mostly plants."

The best way to follow that advice would be the Mediterranean diet, which is really not a "diet" at all. Think of how they eat in Greece, Italy, France, and Spain (or at least used to eat, before Westernization and the importation of highly processed foods): lots of fruits, vegetables, grains (mostly whole), olive oil, beans, nuts, legumes, seeds, herbs, and spices. Every meal should include these foods as a base. At least twice a week, eat fresh fish and seafood (not frozen fish sticks or fried catfish). Consume moderate portions of poultry, eggs, cheese, and yogurt. Less often, eat meats—especially red and processed meats—and sweets (i.e., no more than a few times a month). Replace butter with healthy fats, such as olive oil. Limit salt and sugar. If you want to drink red wine in moderation, that's cool, but it's optional. Yes, fresh strawberries don't have the same flavor burst or mouthfeel as Skittles, but they do offer a much greater return on investment. The research supports that.

If someone else (a restaurant or a factory) is preparing your meal, odds are that the meal/product is not very healthy. There are certainly exceptions to the rule, but they still are exceptions. Your health and nutrition goals are not aligned with their goals—or at least they shouldn't be. *You* want to provide outstanding fuel for your body so you can think clearly, feel and look great, sleep better, have plenty of energy, and avoid illness. *They* want what's in your wallet. Period. Their objective is to keep cost of goods low, keep margins high, and produce a product that you simply can't say no to. If they can do all of that, the odds are high that you will regularly come back for more.

Don't let them win the battle! Start by simply asking, "What will this food or beverage choice do for me? Will it really fuel me, or simply satisfy a craving for something sweet and/or salty? Am I eating because I'm hungry, or am I eating out of habit or because

I'm bored, lonely, or sad?" Many of us were often told as kids to clean our plates because "there are starving children in China." I'm not sure why, but I never considered asking how eating the food on my plate would have any impact on kids on the other side of the planet.

Remember, you don't have to be perfect at every meal of every day, but it's important to realize you can't buy health; you have to earn it. Your body really wants to be healthy. It's designed to be healthy. Don't succumb to the Evil Empire and allow huge for-profit corporations to manipulate what you put in your mouth. Invest in yourself, and if you have them, invest in your children and grandchildren.

"Man is what he eats."
– Ludwig Feuerbach

"Never give up on something that you can't go a day
without thinking about."
– Winston Churchill

10.

What Are We Talking About?

When people find out what I do for a living, they often inquire, "Can I ask you a question about nutrition?"

I always respond with a question of my own: "Are we talking about *weight,* or are we talking about *health*?" From my perspective, these are two very distinct discussions. First, let's talk about weight. Close to three out of four American adults are either overweight (BMI of 25–29) or obese (BMI >30). Many of them have been trying for years—perhaps decades—to lose weight and, more important, keep it off. If you're in this category, don't worry: You're obviously not alone. You might be surprised to hear why you've not had much success.

(*Full disclosure*: My company, ACAP Health, distributes a weight-loss and MetS intervention program known as Naturally Slim (www.naturallyslim.com). It's used by companies, hospitals, universities, cities, counties, and states all over the country and has helped hundreds of thousands of individuals lose weight and keep it off. The reason I share this is that we have years of experience, overwhelming longitudinal data, and peer-reviewed evidence to support what I'm about to share with you. When it comes to weight loss, for the most part, *what* you eat is not as important as *when* and *how* you eat. It's true. Marcia Upson, a family nurse practitioner whose mother developed the original Naturally Slim program, has shared this mantra for years. And guess what? Most people don't want to believe it. For some reason, the majority of individuals think they have to eat only certain foods or certain macronutrients in order to lose weight, but the data do not support that *at all*.)

The only way to enjoy sustainable weight loss is to build skills that allow you to permanently change your behavior around food. It's not the food itself; it's simply how you behave around food that makes a difference, from a weight perspective. This contention is supported by multiple large, well-controlled clinical trials, including the Diabetes Prevention Program (DPP), Pounds Lost, and Look Ahead.

What Gives?

Ever wonder why certain people seem to maintain a healthy weight with what appears to be no effort at all? They don't eat salads every time they go out to restaurants. They don't count calories, weigh their food, or add up points. They may or may not exercise. They simply eat what they want and maintain a normal, healthy weight. We used to think these people had a fast metabolism or were somehow genetically blessed. We know now, however, that with very few exceptions, that's not the case. They just employ, without much effort, certain behaviors that allow them to enjoy the foods they love, in appropriate portions, and not gain weight. The good news is, with some intentional effort, everyone can learn these skills and turn them into habits.

Now I know, based on several years of experience, there's a very strong chance that right now you're thinking, *this guy has lost his mind.* I get it, I really do. I understand that for years and years, we've been taught certain things that *must* happen for us to lose weight. Obviously, those things are not working, because collectively, our country is the heaviest it's ever been. You *can* lose weight even while eating pizza, barbeque, hamburgers, or Mexican food. I promise. In the process, your metabolic risk factors will also improve, which will lower your risk of dangerous conditions such as diabetes, heart disease, stroke, and dementia.

The most important step for permanent weight loss is learning to eat when you're hungry and not when you're not. This seems pretty intuitive, but most folks eat robotically, based on the time on the clock—that is in some variation, breakfast at 7:00, lunch at noon, dinner at 6:00. Understand that hunger is not binary; it's a continuum. You must learn to listen to your hunger signals (which requires learning the difference between *appetite* and *hunger*) and then eat at the appropriate time. This can vary pretty dramatically from person to person. If you eat too soon or too late, it will be impossible for you to lose weight.

Breakfast: To Eat or Not to Eat?

This brings up the topic of breakfast. The common belief is that eating breakfast is mandatory for weight loss. I hear it all the time: "Breakfast jumpstarts the metabolism, so you have to start the day by eating a good breakfast." Please hear me when I say this: Breakfast is *not* essential for weight loss. If you are actually hungry early in the morning, by all means, eat breakfast; however, many people confuse thirst for hunger and end up eating when they really don't need to. Whether you eat breakfast or not, it's not a bad idea to start your day with a big glass of water. When you wake up in the morning, you've just spent (I hope) at least seven hours sleeping. During that time, you lost fluid by respirating (breathing) and perspiring (to at least some degree), then you urinated as soon as you got up. That adds up to a lot of dehydration, so starting the day with a glass of water helps to replace much of that lost fluid. About 57–60 percent of your body is water, so don't try to run on a depleted tank.

If you are still convinced that breakfast is essential for weight loss, I encourage you to review the results of a large study published in *Physiology and Behavior* in 2015 ("Effect of Skipping Breakfast on Subsequent Energy Intake"). In this study, researchers at Cornell University followed a group of adults to determine whether skipping breakfast had any effect on overall caloric consumption. As it turned out, breakfast skippers consumed 408 *fewer* calories per day than those who chowed down first thing in the morning.

"If you skip breakfast," the researchers noted, "you may be hungrier, but you won't eat enough calories to make up for the lost breakfast." Now, just to be clear, I'm *not* saying don't eat breakfast if you want to lose weight. What I *am* saying is learn to eat when you are truly hungry and not just because of a lifelong routine.

Slow down, and Beware of Sugar

Another key to successful, permanent weight loss is to *slow down*. It takes twenty to thirty minutes for your stomach to tell your brain when it's had enough, but because of our hectic, overbooked, stressed-out lifestyles, we often take fewer than ten minutes to eat a meal. Europeans are horrified when they visit the United States and see how fast Americans consume our food. If you take the time to enjoy and savor the foods you truly desire, you will find that you're completely satisfied and that you got there on far less food than you thought was necessary. Successful weight loss is not about knowledge. As my friend and colleague Dr. Tim Church likes to say, "Ask any heavy person how many calories are in a muffin and they'll tell you . . . but they'll still eat the muffin!" Knowledge alone does not change behavior. We must learn the proper skills if we are serious about permanent weight loss.

One final note: When I say you can eat whatever foods you want, the one thing you *must* keep an eye on is sugar. Sugar is added to all sorts of processed foods and is virtually omnipresent in the standard American diet, often referred to as the SAD diet. The majority of the sugar that Americans consume does not come out of the sugar bowl. It's added in all sorts of clever ways by the big food companies because they know it drives craveability. It makes good business sense for them, but it makes no sense for you—especially if you want to lose weight.

> "Hara hachi bu... (Eat until you are 80% full.")
> – Confucius

"Don't be afraid to go out on a limb.
That's where the fruit is."
– H. Jackson Browne

11.

That's Just Nuts:
The Benefits of Nuts, Seeds, and Legumes

As I've written throughout this book, food is fuel. Just like a car needs gasoline to run, humans need food to live—not just to breathe, but to flourish. As I've mentioned before, the *quantity* of food is obviously important, but so is the *quality*. Many Americans overlook the importance of quality of their diets. In terms of quantity, we measure food in calories. Humans require a certain amount of calories every day to satisfy such basic needs as keeping the heart, lungs, and brain operating. This number of calories is known as your resting metabolic rate (RMR). You can have your RMR measured with a simple breath test that many dieticians offer for around a hundred bucks.

Your caloric needs go up as you increase your physical activity levels, just as your car requires more gasoline to drive from Dallas to New York than it does to drive from Dallas to Fort Worth. When the topic of weight loss is discussed, you often hear that "a calorie is a calorie," whether that calorie comes from a soft drink or a lentil. Basically, that's true, and if you eat more calories than you burn, you gain weight, and if you burn more calories than you eat, you lose weight. However, not all calories are created equal. Some calories last longer than others; they provide better *mileage,* also known as *satiety.* Take, for instance, nuts. Even though nuts are relatively high in calories, they are quite good for us and they make us feel full longer. Nuts are high in fat (heart-healthy unsaturated fat) and are a solid source of protein and fiber—all of which help increase satiety. Certain foods, like nuts, increase satiety, while others tend to decrease our sense of fullness. If you are looking to lose or maintain weight, satiety is crucial. If you feel full (i.e., not hungry), you are generally not motivated to eat.

Nuts and Satiety

In 2003, the US Food and Drug Administration issued a qualified health claim regarding nuts: "Scientific evidence suggests but does not prove that eating 1.5 ounces per day of most nuts, as part of a diet low in saturated fat and cholesterol, may reduce the risk of heart disease." Nuts eligible in this claim include almonds, hazelnuts, peanuts (although they are technically legumes), pecans, some pine nuts, pistachios, and walnuts.

Nuts also provide many minerals important for the body's optimal function, including magnesium, manganese, zinc, and phosphorus. The National Heart, Lung, and Blood Institute, as part of their well-known DASH (Dietary Approaches to Stop Hypertension) diet, recommends four to five servings per week from the nuts, seeds, and legumes (peanuts, dried beans, lentils, and peas) category. These foods may help lower blood pressure and reduce the risk of stroke.

Portion Control Is Key

The crucial point is not to eat too many nuts, which sometimes is pretty challenging, especially if the nuts are salted. Nuts are naturally low in salt, but because food providers know that salt increases craveability, they often will add it (salt increases thirst, which is why many bars provide salted nuts as snacks). When shopping, look for unsalted or lightly salted nuts.

Generally, a serving of nuts equals 1.5 ounces (42 grams), or about a third of a cup. Obviously, though, there is a great deal of variety among nuts from caloric, taste, and nutritional perspectives.

Almonds, cashews, pine nuts, and pistachios are the lowest in calories (about 240 calories per 1.5-ounce serving). Pecans, macadamias, and walnuts are on the higher side (about 300 calories per serving). If you are watching your weight, be sure to factor these totals into your food log.

I enjoy nuts as a bridge to help get me from one meal to the next. I keep a container of mixed nuts in my desk at work. If I get a little hungry in between meals, I'll have just a few nuts, and that usually is all I need to get me to the next meal. When traveling, I put about a third of a cup of mixed nuts in a small, resealable snack bag. I toss in a few peanut M&M's for a delicious and filling snack on the go. My main goal is to avoid getting so hungry that I'm forced to select from the limited, usually non-nutritious, options provided at airports or on the plane. I like to make sure that *I*, not the environment (wherever I may be), am the one in charge of my fuel, and nuts are a great way for me to do that.

"Avoid fried foods, which angry up the blood."
– Satchel Paige

"As a child, my family's menu consisted of two choices: take it, or leave it."
– Buddy Hackett

12.

Something to Chew On: Feeding Our Kids

Not long ago, I was on a conference call with a group of ten executives from various Michigan-based companies. We were discussing topics related to both personal and corporate wellness. I had spoken to the group in person six months earlier, and we were reconvening by phone to share what progress had been made.

During the call, one of the executives asked if I thought it was alright for his eleven-year-old son to drink the nutrition shake Ensure, which is often given to elderly people who, for various reasons, have trouble getting enough nutrition through a traditional diet. The gentleman said that the only things his son would eat were chicken nuggets and cereal. I paused for a moment, then asked, "Does your son drive?"

He responded, "No, of course not, he's only eleven."

I queried, "Does he do the grocery shopping in your family?"

Silence. This guy knew where I was going. Here was an intelligent, highly educated business executive admitting that he had no control over what his young son ate. Parents, I implore you: Be parents!

Dr. Tedd Mitchell, former president of Cooper Clinic in Dallas and current president of the Texas Tech Health Sciences Center, is one of the most insightful individuals I have ever met. He is a third-generation doctor who grew up in rural East Texas. He loves to tell the story of the rancher who was standing out in his field one day with his dog and a fellow rancher. The visitor looked down and asked, "What's that your dog's eating?"

"A turnip," came the simple reply.

"A turnip? My dog would *never* eat a turnip!"

This triggered the response: "Neither would mine . . . for the first three days."

The point is simple: No dog (or child) would ever willingly starve to death. Allowing children to dictate a very limited menu selection is not only bad parenting; it's also unhealthy for the child. I get it; kids can be finicky eaters, but that doesn't mean we should give up and serve them only what they demand. The big food companies would certainly love that. They invest many millions of dollars to produce "food" designed to be cheap, convenient, and great-tasting (remember, they engineer the ratio of salt, sugar, and fat)—but that doesn't mean this "food" is nutritious.

As parents, we cannot turn over the health and welfare of our children to companies that are interested only in selling more of their products. Our responsibility is to provide our children with a wide variety of quality nutrients to help them grow and thrive.

A 2010 study out of Northern Michigan University by Amy Ross looked at the link between nutrition and academic performance, specifically examining nutrition and its relationship to brain function, cognition, learning, and social behaviors, as reported in other studies. No doubt about it: There is a direct link between quality of nutrition and level of brain function. Just because a child might scream, pout, and throw a fit does not, in any way, alter our responsibility to provide them with quality nutrition. We are the grown-ups, and we're in charge! Prepare the dinner and serve it to the child. If he or she refuses to eat it, calmly say, "No problem, I'll see you at breakfast." Then stick to it. Don't get into a shouting match or debate. Just let the child know that this is the only option for this meal, and he or she will have another opportunity tomorrow. Let the child go to bed hungry.

Yes, they will test you. And yes, they won't believe you would ever do such a thing. Trust me, if you follow through with this approach, it will take only once or twice before Junior gets the message. You have to be consistent and be willing to stick to your guns, no matter how hard it may get. You may be thinking this is harsh and unrealistic—but it's not, at all. It's the only way your child will ever develop a taste for healthy, nutritious food (maybe even turnips!). Serving children nothing but highly processed, convenient crud is not the solution. It's an easy way out, but it's not in the best interest of your child.

According to the Centers for Disease Control and Prevention, as of 2017, 18.5 percent of children are obese. That is a 34 percent increase since 2000! Childhood obesity has immediate and long-term effects on health and well-being, including increasing risk factors for cardiovascular disease (e.g., high cholesterol and high blood pressure), bone and joint problems, sleep apnea, and social and psychological issues (e.g., stigmatization and poor self-esteem). And obese children and adolescents are likely to become obese adults, who in turn have increased risk of developing heart disease, type 2 diabetes, stroke, and several types of cancer (e.g., breast, colon, esophagus, kidney, pancreas, multiple myeloma, and Hodgkin's lymphoma). Parents, I implore you to do the right thing and promote healthy lifestyle habits for your children! Their future depends on it.

"Ask yourself what is really important and then have the courage to build your life around the answer."

"If a million people say a foolish thing,
it is still a foolish thing."
– Anatole France

13.

Weight Loss and Metabolic Adaptation

Back in 1958, Dr. Max Wishofsky developed what came to be known as Wishofsky's rule, which states that 3,500 calories equal one pound of body weight. In other words, if you want to lose one pound of weight, you need to burn 3,500 more calories than you consume. This made for simple math. For instance, if you ate five hundred fewer calories than you burned every day for a week, you would lose one pound of body weight (7 days x 500 calories per day = 3,500 calories, or one pound of weight loss).

This rule is basically universal. It's cited in more than 35,000 websites as well as in textbooks, scientific articles, and expert guidelines (including those from the US Surgeon General). Here's the only problem: The Wishofsky Rule doesn't work all of the time. In fact, it seems to be only about half right, as we've learned, with research tools and data that are vastly different than those available in 1958. The 3,500-calorie rule does not take into account age, height, weight, body composition, and physical activity. As it turns out, weight loss is *really* complicated. There is no such thing as one size fits all.

Something called *metabolic adaptation* appears to play a big role in weight loss. In essence, as you lose weight, your basal metabolic rate changes, meaning you don't need as many calories every day just to exist. As you lose more weight, the number of calories needed to maintain your weight also goes down. The result is that weight loss is rarely linear; it's actually curvilinear. Let me explain: Most individuals entering a weight-loss program tend to lose more weight in the first few weeks than they do as time goes on. Over time, additional weight loss becomes more challenging. If you're looking to lose weight, this is not the kind of news you want to hear, but my goal is to give you the truth, not to provide false promises.

This new concept of weight loss is known as the dynamic model. Much of the research on this model has been done by Dr. D. M. Thomas at Montclair State University. There are many free downloadable applications of the dynamic model online, housed in Microsoft Excel and Java platforms. My favorite is the "Single Subject Weight Change Predictor" from the Pennington Biomedical Research Center at Louisiana State University (available at www.pbrc.edu/sswcp). If you enter your baseline age, height, gender, weight, duration of the intervention (a timeline, if you have one), and target caloric intake, the app will provide you with dynamic predictions of weekly weight change. This is a free research tool, so don't expect a slick website with all sorts of bells and whistles. It's pretty basic, but it will provide you with realistic expectations based on solid, credible science. If you are a science geek like me, read the article "Can a Weight Loss of One Pound a Week Be Achieved with a 3500-kcal Deficit?" in the December 2013 issue of *International Journal of Obesity*.

If losing weight is your goal, counting and obsessing over calories is most likely not going to lead to success—not to mention, it's not a very enjoyable way to live. As I mentioned earlier in the book, the research indicates that building skills is the key to sustainable weight loss!

"Truth is not diminished by the number of people that believe it."

"If you have a body, you are an athlete!"
– Bill Bowerman

14.

Finding Your Inner Athlete

Coach Bowerman, the legendary track coach at the University of Oregon, was absolutely right; whether you see yourself as an athlete or not, you, as a human, were designed to move. Experts say we have somewhere between sixty trillion and one hundred trillion (yes, *trillion*!) cells in our bodies, and *every single one* is positively affected when we're physically active. There are benefits for your muscles, lungs, heart, diaphragm, brain, kidney, stomach and intestines, and even your eyes and skin.

Pete Egoscue, a pain-mitigation expert in Del Mar, California, says we are "beautifully designed to run and jump and play and fall and dance, but the problem is most Americans don't do much of that anymore." The truth is, we sit. We sit at work and stare at screens and type on keyboards. We sit in cars. We sit at restaurants. At home, we also sit. We stare at screens on TVs, laptops, desktops, phones, tablets, or other rectangular things. Sitting is *not* healthy; it's *not* what we were designed to do with our time on this earth (see chapter 6).

We were designed *to move*. Early humans had to run to catch their food (the hunters) or at least walk to pick it (the gatherers). If they didn't move, they didn't eat. Today, we've outsourced our food (our providers are big-box grocery stores or restaurants), and movement has become totally optional, as we have developed drive-thrus for everything and our once-small towns and bustling Main Streets have grown into miles upon miles of suburban sprawl. How many times have you seen someone spend several minutes circling the parking lot, trying to find the space closest to the entrance of the store or mall? They burn all sorts of gas trying to avoid walking—what, maybe a hundred or two hundred extra feet? Come on! It's crazy!

Beloved motivational speaker Zig Ziglar often said that for many people, the idea of exercise "is to fill the tub, take a bath, pull the plug and fight the current!" We shouldn't avoid exercise; we should embrace it! Every step we take has a positive effect on every organ in the body—especially the brain! Even if you've never been on a team, worn a uniform, been in a gym, or lifted a weight, I encourage you to start thinking of yourself as an athlete. Dress the part. Get some cool running or walking shoes, some athletic shorts or sweats, and a shirt that let's everyone know you prioritize physical activity.

You might be asking yourself, "Should I be doing that even if I don't look the part yet?" The answer is *yes*! You won't change your body or improve your health until you change your mind-set. Attitude is everything! Since you've already decided that health is a priority, start acting like it. You're an athlete. Let yourself, and those around you, know that physical activity is a part of your life. This might be a total departure from where you are right now, but that's fine. Change your mojo. Stand up straight, shoulders back, and carry yourself with confidence! Don't wait until you hit your "magic" weight or fit into a certain pant or dress size. Start today. Show up with a new attitude. You're headed in a positive direction. Every step—*literally* every step—you take helps you improve.

The human body is beautifully designed. It will do exactly what you ask it to do. Start where you are, not where you used to be or where you think you should be. Know that you are far more capable than you ever imagined. Get moving!

"Life is like a ten-speed bicycle.
Most of us have gears we never use."
– Charles Schultz

"If you had to pick one thing to make people healthier as they age, it would be aerobic exercise."

– James Fries

15.

Cardio Fitness: You Can't Lie to the Treadmill

Dallas's Cooper Institute published an article in the February 5, 2013, issue of the *Annals of Internal Medicine* indicating that men and women who were fit in midlife had a 36 percent lower risk of developing dementia in later life. That's pretty significant. It's well known that being fit lowers the risk of all sorts of things, including heart disease and many cancers. Now the research shows that being fit is also beneficial to the brain, both today and down the road. So, what exactly is fitness, and how much physical activity do you need to achieve and maintain a healthy fitness level?

Fitness is the body's ability to physically work. There are different types of fitness, but the most recognized measurement is something called VO_2 max. This is the body's ability to utilize oxygen during exercise (aka aerobic capacity, often referred to as "cardiovascular fitness"). The higher your VO_2 max, the more fit you are. There is definitely a genetic component to fitness, but just about everyone can improve their fitness level through regular physical activity. The body will do exactly what you ask it to do, as long as you are consistent and patient.

The Treadmill Stress Test

One of the most accepted ways to measure fitness is the maximal treadmill stress test. This test is often used to help determine someone's risk of cardiovascular disease, but one of the side benefits is that it also provides an *objective* measure of fitness. Basically, the longer you can stay on the treadmill, the higher your fitness level. The correlation between someone's treadmill time and their VO_2 max is over 90 percent, which is quite high.

There is a huge difference between *objective data,* like the time someone can stay on a treadmill, and *subjective* data, particularly when it comes to fitness. Asking someone to rate their own fitness level, say on a scale of 1 to 10, would be a subjective assessment, which is seldom accurate. People tell you where they would like to be, where they used to be, where they think you would like them to be, or where they intend to be. Very rarely can folks accurately determine where they are from a fitness perspective.

No matter how you look, what you weigh, or how much you've been exercising, the treadmill test is an objective measure of your current fitness level. It also has a very high retest reliability. That means what you do on the treadmill today will be very close to what you will do tomorrow. There are many protocols used in treadmill testing, but the two most common are the Bruce and Balke protocols. The Balke protocol uses a more gradual increase in elevation (i.e., stress) and is often considered safer, especially for coronary patients. The test starts out innocently enough: You begin walking on a flat treadmill at a pace of 3.3 mph, a fairly comfortable walking speed. After the first minute, the speed stays the same, but the incline increases to 2 percent. No big deal. Then, every minute thereafter, the incline of the treadmill goes up 1 percent while the speed stays steady at 3.3 mph. By increasing the incline, you are increasing the intensity of the activity or workout.

If you are fit enough to stay on the treadmill for twenty-five minutes, the incline will be at 25 percent. That's steep! Clearly, it would be dangerous to continue increasing the incline, so after this point, the speed is increased by 0.2 mph every minute, from 3.3 mph to 3.5, then to 3.7, and so on. Eventually, you won't be able to continue merely walking; you will have to start running, or you will fall off the back of the treadmill. If you've ever tried to run up a 25 percent incline, you know it doesn't take long before you ask yourself, "What in the world am I doing?"

At some point during the treadmill test, whether it's at five minutes or thirty-five minutes, you cry uncle. You reach a point where you can't go any longer. Almost instantly you go from "I've got another minute or so in me" to "I'm *done*!" That time on the treadmill, whatever it is, determines how fit you are. Whoever is administering the test, usually a doctor or an exercise physiologist, will know you're reaching your limit well before you do. He or she watches the monitor for your heart rate and blood pressure, and when these measurements begin to level off, the person administering the test can easily predict how much longer you can go before you hit your wall. Minutes later, after you begin to recover, it's common to say, "You know, I probably could have gone at least another thirty seconds." The odds are against this, but for some reason, it's a common reaction.

How Much Do You Need?

If you want to improve your cardio fitness, you need to have a game plan. The general consensus is that you need to be moderately active for thirty minutes most days of the week. That comes from the U.S. Department of Health and Human Services' recommendation of 150 minutes per week (30 minutes per day x 5 days = 150 minutes). What does it mean to be moderately active? Think of a fairly brisk walk—not jogging, but walking with a purpose (around one hundred steps per minute).

By the way, those thirty minutes do not need to be consecutive. You can do two fifteen-minute bouts, or three ten-minute bouts. Especially if you are just starting out, try ten minutes in the morning before you shower, ten minutes after eating your lunch (which will help get the fuel from your midday meal into your working muscles—especially important if you have issues with blood sugar), then ten minutes after work in the evening. Doing these ten-minute bouts with someone else or while listening to music or a podcast will make the time fly. You won't even know you're exercising.

If you are in better condition and capable of engaging in vigorous activity, you can cut that weekly total from 150 minutes of moderate activity down to just 75 minutes of vigorous activity—think running, swimming, rowing, cycling, and so on. You can probably still carry on a conversation, but you will definitely notice that your heart and lungs are working hard.

If you are just starting out, be sure to get a physical with a health professional, ideally a doctor, to determine if you are ready to begin exercising. Once you have clearance, start gradually. Doing too much too soon will leave you exhausted, sore, and frustrated, which is not safe, fun, or effective. Keep the big picture in mind: You didn't get out of shape overnight, and you're not going to get *in* shape overnight, either. Think of the long term and be patient.

If you've been completely sedentary for a prolonged period of time, I highly encourage you to start with five-minute increments. This suggestion is for your mind rather than for your body. Here's why: For someone who is a regular exerciser, thirty minutes is not that big a deal, but for someone who has been "doing nothing" for a long time, the idea of carving out thirty minutes seems like climbing Mount Everest; it's more of a mental hurdle than a physical one. You may think you're too busy to find thirty minutes in your already overscheduled day. You and I both know that's not really the issue, but this excuse can become an enormous hurdle that keeps you from even starting.

Will you get substantial benefit from a five-minute walk? Not necessarily—at least not physically—but it *will* help you start feeling *capable*. And feeling capable is very important when it comes to behavior change. Once you feel capable of doing five minutes, it's pretty easy to expand that behavior to ten minutes, then twenty, then thirty, and so on. Until you believe you are capable, you will have difficulty getting your body to do what you want it to. As they say, a journey of ten thousand miles begins with just one step. Taking that first step is huge, and it will only happen when you feel capable of success.

Once you start exercising, remember that there are three ways you can alter your workouts; just remember the three "dials" of the acronym FIT, which can be adjusted to alter the workout routine. "F" stands for *frequency,* or how often you are doing the particular activity (once a week? twice a week? seven days a week?). "I" stands for *intensity,* or how hard the activity is. The "T" stands for *time,* or duration. Doing a particular activity for one minute will obviously have a different impact on your physiology and fitness than if you do the same activity for thirty minutes or for three hours.

The key takeaway is simple: How fit you are—that is, how long you stay on the treadmill—is a great predictor of how long you will live. A 2010 study of nearly 1,800 men and women, conducted by Dr, Jarett Berry, found that if you are fit in mid-life, you double your chance to surviving to the age of 85. Conversely, if you are not fit in your 50s, your projected life span is eight years shorter. Cardio fitness trumps just about all other measures of health. Remember, whether you think so or not, you were born to be active—maybe not as a competitive athlete, but definitely as an energetic, functional, strong, capable human being. Don't let the conveniences of the modern world—cars, scooters, moving walkways, escalators, elevators, drive-thru lanes, mobile phones, remote controls, and garage door openers—keep you from using your body the way it was intended. Your priorities are defined by what you can do, not what you say.

You have been given a beautiful gift. Don't take it for granted. Just about everyone can improve his or her fitness level. Remember to start where you are and to be consistent, and before long, you will be amazed at how well your body responds. As Joan Welsh once said:

"A man's health can be judged by what he takes two at a time—pills or stairs."

> "Those who have not time for bodily exercise will sooner or later have to find time for illness."
> – Edward Stanley

16.

Hey, Weight a Minute!
The Benefits of Strength Training

I'm a big fan of the word "strong." It almost always has a positive connotation (except when it precedes the word "odor"). Being strong—physically, mentally, and emotionally—is a good thing. What's interesting is that when people get stronger physically, they also often become stronger mentally and emotionally. That must have something to do with the whole mind-body-spirit connection.

The best way to get physically stronger is to lift weights, or to perform what's called weight-bearing exercise, resistance training or strength training. If you've never "lifted" before, it can be somewhat intimidating. Don't be intimidated. Try it; I guarantee you'll like it! Or at least your *body* will.

If you are an adult and aren't doing some sort of strength training regularly, you are weaker today than you were yesterday. The loss in strength might not be perceivable, since it is gradual, but it's an inescapable reality. It's a fact. Your bones are weaker, too, and you're not as stable, which makes you more susceptible to falls and fractures as you age. The expression "use it or lose it" applies to strength. As we get older, we all lose muscle mass. The technical term for that is sarcopenia (muscle wasting). Weight training slows and actually reverses that process. The great news is that effective strength training doesn't take that much time; it just takes consistency: about twenty minutes per workout (as long as you know what you are doing) two to three times per week.

Not Just for Men

Some women are hesitant to lift weights, fearing they will begin to look too bulky and lose their feminine appearance. Trust me, that fear is unfounded; you are not going to look like "Ahh-nold." Regular weight training helps to trim and contour the body, helps prevent weight gain, and supports weight loss maintenance. Proper weight training can help improve posture and body image, so please don't avoid it. Embrace it! It's never too late to start, and measurable results can happen at any age.

Miriam Nelson, a researcher at Tufts University, has done fascinating research with women in their eighties and nineties that shows a correlation between weight training and increases in strength and bone density. Her research reveals a lowered risk of osteoporosis, osteopenia (pre-osteoporosis), and bone fractures. You can read about these studies in Dr. Nelson's book *Strong Women, Strong Bones*, published in 2000. She also maintains an excellent website at www.strongwomen.com, with the mission of "lifting women to better health." (By the way, these improvements apply to men, as well.)

Other benefits from strength training include improved glucose metabolism, blood lipid levels, and blood pressure values. Weight-bearing exercise helps with maintenance of structural integrity of the head, neck, spine, and pelvis. From a functional standpoint, if you improve your strength, you'll find it easier to move, lift, and carry things, in all areas of your life. If you're a golfer, you'll become "longer" off the tee; if you play softball, you'll find it easier to "go yard." Maybe most important, if you're a parent, grandparent, or even great-grandparent, you'll be able to play with the kids rather than just watch them play. They will appreciate that as much as you do.

As with all exercise, it's critical to start where you are. If you have never lifted weights before, or if it's been years since your last workout, begin gradually and do not go overboard! If you do too much too soon, you will become very sore and most likely will quit long before you have a chance to see any improvement. Be patient. The results can be significant, but you have to progress gradually and follow a well-constructed plan. Be especially careful if you start some sort of high-intensity commercial routine like P90-X, Insanity, Boot Camp, CrossFit, and so on. It's tempting to emulate the routines of individuals who already are in outstanding shape, but be warned: This will quickly lead to frustration and injury. Start where *you* are!

Consult the Experts

I encourage you to be willing to trust the expertise of professionals. Talk with your doctor or a certified fitness pro for advice on how to get started. Find a personal trainer to help you begin with a simple weight-bearing regimen, or if you are already working out, ask him or her to take you to the next level. It's well worth the investment. You don't need to use a trainer for every workout, and you don't need to join a gym in order to hire one. Many trainers will come to your home or a local park and will customize a workout plan based on your goals and what equipment you already own. If you know what you're doing, it doesn't take a lot of expensive equipment to perform strength training. With a couple of dumbbells, a resistance band, and a stability ball, you can achieve an amazing full-body workout.

As with any other professionals, not all personal trainers are created equal. Seek out someone with experience who has a four-year degree in some sort of exercise science like kinesiology or exercise physiology. Additional credentials and certifications from recognized organizations are also important (look for ACSM, NSCA, NASM, and PTA Global).

When you begin a weight-training routine, you will *get* stronger long before you *look* stronger. What actually occurs is that your nervous system becomes more efficient at recruiting muscle fiber, which translates into increased strength (i.e., you are able to lift more weight than when you started). It's natural to look in the mirror and expect to see a chiseled, more defined physique, but those visible changes come with time. Give yourself at least eight weeks of consistent training before you can expect to see any substantial physical transformation. Trust me, it will happen, especially if you are combining your training with healthy nutrition and a cardio fitness routine.

If you've never considered strength training before, I enthusiastically encourage you to do so. Not everyone will enjoy the process as much as others, but I've heard time and time again how getting stronger has made a difference in someone's health, both physically and mentally. Studies indicate that if you are told what to expect with any new behavior, you are much more likely to stick with it and form a new habit, so I'm telling you now: As long as you're patient and consistent, you'll enjoy significant measurable improvement. Weight training will help you *today* with increased strength, balance, energy, and confidence, but it will also help you in the *years to come*. It's a wonderfully beneficial activity that will dramatically increase your odds of being independent, functional, and productive as you age.

"The doctor of the future will give no medicine,
but will invest his patients in the care of the human
frame, in diet and in the cause and prevention
of disease."
– Thomas Edison

"We don't stop playing because we grow old;
we grow old because we stop playing."
– George Bernard Shaw

17.

The Best Time of Day to Exercise

I am often asked when is the best time of day to exercise. My standard reply is "The best time for you to exercise is when you *will* exercise." You can do just about anything for a short while—even a high-intensity boot camp class at five a.m.—but if the addition is too disruptive to your normal routine, it probably won't be sustainable. If you really want to develop an exercise habit that will last a lifetime, you need to be strategic. Identify a time of day when exercise is most likely to happen for you. Your best time might be completely different than mine, which happens to be at lunch during the week and in mornings or late afternoons on the weekends.

We are all different. We have different jobs, schedules, rhythms (some of us are morning people, others not so much), commitments, obligations, opportunities, and so on. If you like to exercise in a group setting and are motivated by a surrounding community of exercisers, obviously, your options will be limited to when classes are offered. If you work out with a buddy or buddies, you'll have to coordinate schedules. If you have young kids, mornings might not work at all because you have to help them get ready and off to school. During the week, I usually work out at lunch because that's when it's easiest for me. Easy is good. Remember, the more hurdles you must clear, the less likely you are to stick with a new behavior. I prefer to come in to work early because I can beat the traffic and get plenty accomplished before the phone starts ringing. I have it pretty easy: Since there's a fitness center just three floors below my office and a long walking and biking path just across the street, I have plenty of options and no excuses. Around Noon, I grab my gym bag, work out, have a quick shower, then come back to my office and eat lunch while answering e-mails at my desk. (If I had an issue with low blood sugar, I would eat before my workout.)

The culture of my work environment not only permits working out, but actually encourages and incentivizes me to stay active. There are a multitude of benefits from a workout—not the least of which is that my productivity and immunity increase when I'm fit. The latest research shows that exercise can make you happier, smarter, and more energetic. That's just good business.

For other folks, this middle-of-the-day workout wouldn't be at all feasible. Many people prefer to work out first thing in the morning or after work. Some individuals like to work out right before bedtime; this is fine, as long as doing so doesn't negatively affect your ability to go to sleep. For some, working out right before bed actually *helps* them get to sleep. You may need to experiment and find out exactly what makes the most sense for the way you're wired.

The takeaway is to be intentional about how you incorporate a workout into your day. Plan your exercise ahead of time, just like you would a meeting or business lunch. Make exercise a priority, something that is nonnegotiable. Put it on all of your calendars (smartphone, PC, tablet, and so on). Pick a time of day when you know you are least likely to get derailed.

Now, all that said, studies show that the most *consistent* exercisers are those who work out first thing in the morning. As soon as you finish, you can check it off your to-do list and nothing can get in the way. Early-morning exercising is also a terrific way to jump-start the day; You increase your heart rate and blood blow, activate your brain, get the endorphins flowing, and set the stage for a productive day!

> "The elevator to success is out of order.
> You'll have to use the stairs... one at a time."
> – Joe Girard

> "To give anything less than your best
> is to sacrifice the gift."
> – Steve Prefontaine

18.

A Little Pep Talk: Invest in Yourself

I went for a solo bike ride one morning not long ago. Nothing too crazy—just over twenty miles, about an hour and twenty minutes of cardio endurance. It was summer in Texas, so, no surprise, it was warm, but there was a pleasant, mild breeze. During a long straightaway, I was passed by a car that had a "0.0" sticker on the back window. I find those pretty funny. I'm sure you've seen the 13.1, 26.2, 70.3, and 140.6 stickers. They let the world know what kind of athlete you are: half-marathoner (13.1 miles), marathoner (26.2 miles), half-Ironman triathlete (1.2-mile swim, 56-mile bike, 13.1-mile run), or full Ironman (2.4-mile swim, 112-mile ride, 26.2-mile run . . . amazing!). These numbers represent an insider code, a shorthand for extreme endurance athletes.

The "0.0" sticker announces to the world, "I'm a couch potato and proud of it!" It also might be sending this message: "Hey, all you self-absorbed wannabes, get over yourselves!" There is an enormous difference between a "0.0" and a "140.6." Although I certainly admire and respect anyone who has done a full Ironman, I know that if your goal is to improve your health and immunity, lower your risk of chronic disease (including dementia and Alzheimer's), sleep better, feel better, look better, love better, manage stress, have more energy, and push back the onset of disability, then you don't have to spend hours upon hours in the water, on a bike, or running on a trail, street, or treadmill. Basically, you simply need to get off the couch regularly! Walk the dog, even if you don't have one!

Staying Fit: The Hidden Benefits

I spend a great deal of time on the road. While waiting for a recent a flight, I was blown away by the number of individuals having problems walking through the airport. Simply walking. They were expending incredible effort just to walk a couple of hundred feet between gates. It was painful to watch but, I suspect, much more painful to experience. It made me sad, especially because many of these people looked to be in their twenties and thirties—way too young to be struggling like that.

This morning on my bike ride, I thought about all the benefits I was receiving. First, my heart rate was elevated and blood was flowing at a faster rate than if I were sitting at home, reading the paper or staring at my phone. Endurance, or aerobic, exercise has hundreds of benefits, but one I tend to concentrate on is something called collateral circulation. When you stress the cardiovascular system regularly through exercise, in essence, you grow more blood vessels and increase the options to get blood from point A to point B. That means if one vessel becomes clogged or occluded, there are alternative pathways to bypass the congestion. I think about this benefit often because my father died from heart disease. As my heart ages, I'd like it to have as many alternative routes as possible.

My heart is not the only organ receiving benefit during my bike rides, however. Several large muscle groups, including my quads and hamstrings (the front and back muscles of the thighs) and calves were being challenged—not so much that they burned, but just enough to let me know they were working. By pushing myself a bit, I was sending a message to those muscles to get stronger. Because the body responds to stress by adapting, this extra effort means I was helping to maintain my strength. Staying strong is important to me. I have twin grandsons. My goal is simple: I want to *play* with them, not just *watch* them play.

My legs weren't the only things working hard during the morning ride, either. My back, abs, and triceps were also engaged, so I was getting a great overall workout. Again, nothing crazy—just enough to feel alive.

In addition to all the muscle benefit, I was breathing fresh air, enjoying the scenery, and working up a sweat. Sweating is your body's way of releasing excess heat, and sweating during moderate to vigorous exercise is a much better way to remove toxins from the body than is an ill-advised "cleanse."

Another benefit of the ride was that I soaked in a bit of vitamin D, although it was still early and there wasn't much UVB light yet. (The longer your shadow, the lower the amount of UVB light available.) UVB is what triggers the synthesis of vitamin D in the body.

Walking Works, Too!

When I finished my ride, I felt great. I had just spent eighty minutes setting the stage for the day. I was back home before 9:30 and had already amassed the equivalent of more than ten thousand steps. For those of you with "wearables" (Fitbits, Fuel Bands, Vivofits, and others), according to Dr. Catrine Tudor-Locke (an associate dean for research as well as a professor and department chair at the University of Massachusetts–Amherst who has done extensive research on walking behaviors), the true benefit of activity begins at 7,500 steps per day, not the 10,000 that everyone assumes is the magic number. More is always better, but benefit begins at 7,500.

So, for the guy who passed me with the "0.0" sticker, I get it! There are plenty of folks who don't like to exercise. There are also plenty of people who are tired, hurt, depressed, and struggling just to get through the day—or from gate to gate at the airport. All I'm suggesting is that the only person who can improve your health is you. The answer is not a pill or a procedure. You were born to move—to run, jump, play, fall, and dance—all the things we used to do when we were young—when we were, as walking advocate Mark Fenton puts it, "free-range kids."

Sure, you can get through life avoiding physical activity, but you aren't going to thrive. You aren't going to be able to take advantage of all the great things the world has to offer. Regular, consistent physical activity (aka exercise) is the single best investment you can make in yourself. You don't have to join a gym, buy an expensive bike, or spend a bunch of money on all sorts of shoes, clothing, or equipment. You just need to move!

> "Life is like riding a bicycle.
> You don't fall off unless you stop pedaling."
> – Claude D. Pepper

PART 3

Looking Downfield

"If you are not making someone's life better,
you are wasting your time."

19.

What's Your Why?
Finding Motivation That Sustains You

Motivation is an interesting concept. Many behavioral experts, including B. J. Fogg at Stanford University, claim that it's very hard to stay motivated over a prolonged period of time. Motivation has a tendency to ebb and flow. I agree you can't stay permanently "pumped up," but I think that if you take the time to really dig deep and practice some introspection, it can make a big difference in influencing how you live daily. Finding your *why* might provide a boost that can mean the difference between hitting the snooze button and hitting the gym.

Neither of my parents was at all athletic. Even though they didn't prod me, I started playing baseball in third grade, basketball in fourth grade, and football in sixth grade. I absolutely loved playing sports. There weren't many days I wasn't playing something, whether it was organized games, practice, or just pickup. I was an only child, so I found my "brothers" on the playground or in the gym.

My mom and dad split up when I was eight. Whenever I went to visit my dad on weekends, I would take my glove or a ball, hoping that he might want to play catch or shoot some hoops, but that rarely happened. He just wasn't interested. Because of his crazy schedule as an airline pilot, he was often tired and preferred to take naps rather than play anything.

I promised myself that if I ever had kids, and if they wanted to play, I would never say no. My wife and I have been blessed with two terrific children, Lauren and Andrew, although neither one of them are kids anymore. While Lauren and I share a passion for music, Andrew has always loved sports. If it involved keeping score, he was interested, which certainly didn't break my heart. From the time he could walk, Andrew and I were kicking or bouncing a ball, playing chase, or wrestling (often to the chagrin of his mother and sister). Andrew was a typical boy, and I made a strong effort to be a willing participant in whatever sport was in season—as a teammate, opponent, or coach. That commitment continues today.

My Why: Staying Ready

A few years ago, I flew to Las Vegas for a speaking engagement. It was a Wednesday afternoon. The gentleman sitting next to me on the plane noticed a Dallas Marathon logo on my watch, and we started chatting about running. Turns out, he worked for BNSF Railway—a huge company that employs several former collegiate runners. Just about every year, the company team wins the five-person relay at the Dallas Marathon in December—and not by a little! This guy was one of those runners. He had attended the University of North Texas and ran a 4:11 mile. If you're a nonrunner, let me assure you, that is freakishly fast!

As we talked, I learned that on the upcoming Saturday, this guy and his coworker (another one of the gazelles) were competing in the Original Mud Run in Fort Worth. The event, a 10K (6.2 mile) race, included about twenty obstacles, most of which involved mud and/or water, walls, and ropes. Competitors run, climb, swing, jump, swim, and crawl their way through the course, which hugs the bank of the Trinity River. Oh yeah, participants are encouraged to wear camo pants and boots. Think Navy Seal or Green Beret gear.

I was intrigued. The second I got to my hotel, I did some online research. The pictures of previous races were awesome! It was a third-grade boy's dream come true—playing in mud and water and not worrying about how dirty you got! How cool is that? In fact, the muddier, the better. They even had a big fire truck in the parking lot to hose you down after you finished. I immediately sent Andrew a text encouraging him to check out the website. At the time, he was a junior at Texas Christian University in Fort Worth, and I suspected this might be right up his alley.

Within five minutes, I got the reply: "I'm in!" I thought, with a broad smile, *oh crap, what have I got myself into?* By now, it was Wednesday night. The race was Saturday morning, three days away! No worries. I faxed in our entry forms (along with a very long insurance waiver), went to Big Five Sporting Goods in Las Vegas to get my fatigues, and called my son to start planning our strategy. I was fifty-four at the time; Andrew was twenty-one. Obviously, neither one of us had time to train for the event, but we talked about how we would run it together and what a blast we anticipated having.

On race day, we arrived early to make sure we had time to check in and scout out the course. There were all sorts of competitors—men and women, young and old, many dressed as if they were ready to invade Normandy. Because of the size of the field, participants started in assigned flights. I'll admit, before they fired the start gun, I was a tad nervous. What if this thing was a lot tougher than I imagined? My concern was quickly alleviated. Within the first half mile, I knew this event was going to be a ball. One of the first obstacles was crossing the Trinity River via a rope secured to the opposite bank. It was October and the water was brisk, but Andrew and I are pretty strong swimmers. Despite wearing long pants, it wasn't too much of a problem.

Shortly after emerging soaking wet from the Trinity, we had to shimmy on our bellies about forty yards in thick, slick, viscous mud, all the while making sure not to lift up too high because we were under a barbwire canopy about eighteen inches off the ground. It turns out that sharp barbwire can be *very* motivating!

After every obstacle, we would run a while, then hit another obstacle. Then we would run some more. We had to climb over walls, swing on monkey bars to clear mud pools, cross the river three more times, traverse waist-deep swamps, and scale a rickety trellis at least thirty feet high (the last obstacle)! At least two or three times during the almost-two-hour thrill-seeking adventure, Andrew laughed and exclaimed, "This is the coolest thing we've ever done!" We pushed ourselves hard, but we loved every minute of it, and we crossed the finish line together. What a great memory!

This experience with my son helps to explain my *why*—why I'm motivated to *stay* in shape. I want to stay ready. Always. Ready to do Mud Runs at the drop of a hat with Andrew. Ready to play chase with my grandsons, Henry and Hudson. Ready to hike down the Grand Canyon or up to Cloud's Rest in Yosemite with members of my executive leadership group. Ready to do a half marathon or sprint triathlon with friends and colleagues. My days of hoping to actually win an event are long gone, but I want to participate for as long as possible!

Discover Your Drive

You may have no intention of ever doing a Mud Run, and that's certainly fine, but I bet there's something you enjoy doing and your life would be much more fulfilling if you could do this activity for as long as possible. Maybe it's getting on the floor and playing with your kids, grandkids, or, dare I say it, great-grandkids. Maybe it's visiting a foreign city and wandering for hours through museums and shops without feeling exhausted. What about gardening? Riding bikes? Touring the country by motorcycle? Dancing? You don't need to be an elite athlete. You don't need to climb mountains. You just need to get off the couch! Get muddy! Walk the darn dog, even if you don't have one! Don't limit yourself. Stay ready!

As my good friend Bill Case says, "You must be present to win!" That's the way life works. You gotta stay ready. You have to *show up*. Don't be a spectator. Get *in* the game, whatever the game happens to be. Take some time and really think about what your life will be like in five, ten, twenty-five, even fifty years from today. What's your default future? Will it be filled with incredible events and adventures with your family and friends, or will it be in an assisted-living facility with some stranger wheeling you to the dining hall?

Rest assured, you are not treading water. One month from now, you will be either healthier or less healthy than you are today. Your stock is either going up or down. What's it going to be? All data prove, without a shadow of a doubt, that your habits and environment (i.e., lifestyle choices) play an enormous role in your future, in your quality of life. No one can embrace healthy habits for you. No one has more impact on your health and future than you do. You cannot outsource your health. Discover your *why*, and maybe it will help you avoid the snooze button!

> "Knowing your sense of purpose is worth up to seven years of extra life expectancy."
> – Dan Buettner

"Whoever I am or whatever I am doing, some kind of
excellence is within my reach."
– John W. Gardner

20.

Time Is Not the Problem!

I love having "what if" discussions with Dr. Tim Church, my good friend and colleague at ACAP Health. Tim has lots of impressive letters after his name (MD, PhD, MPH), and he rarely lacks for an opinion, so our conversations often become fairly spirited debates, but there is one question on which Tim and I are in complete agreement: If someone could do only *one thing* to improve their health, looking downfield, what would it be? Obviously, there are all sorts of possibilities: eat healthier, lose weight, stop smoking, drink more water, get more sleep, improve fitness, take vitamin D and omega-3 supplements, consistently wash your hands, floss, manage stress, stretch regularly, practice yoga or Pilates, spend more time with family and friends, take prescribed medications properly and so on. All of these directives would have a positive impact on an individual's health, but what is the single most effective thing?

The answer: improve fitness. Plenty of data support this position, so let's not get wrapped around the axle. The next relevant question is, of course, how does one improve their fitness level? You already know the deceptively simple answer: exercise. Yes, that word that is dreaded and cringe-worthy for so many folks. Even though humans were created to move beautifully, physical activity has become completely optional. We *can't* live very long without food and sleep. We *can* live without exercise.

But we can't live well.

Improving one's fitness through physical activity has a hugely positive impact on both the length and quality of life. I contend that the vast majority of humans are driven by the desire to look and feel better, and there's no question that exercise helps you meet both of those goals.

Weekly Recommendations

Unfortunately, the research clearly shows most folks are falling short of the weekly recommendations for exercise. We need to be physically active for 30 minutes a day, several days a week. As noted in Chapter 15, here are the actual recommendations for adults from the Department of Health and Human Services:

- 150 minutes per week of moderate-intensity physical activity (i.e., brisk walking) *or;*
- 75 minutes per week of vigorous-intensity physical activity (i.e., running, swimming, cycling, etc.) and;
- At least two sessions per week of strength training (i.e., weight lifting or resistance training) that incorporates all major muscle groups (legs, hips, back, abdomen, chest, shoulders and arms). If you know what you're doing, this should take no more than 20 minutes per session

In all, we're talking somewhere between 115 and 190 minutes of exercise per week. That doesn't seem like too much to ask. There are 168 hours in a week, so 115–190 minutes represent less than two percent of our total available time. Inexplicably, though, when I ask folks why they avoid exercise, the practically universal answer is, "I don't have the time!" I'm sorry, but that's a lousy excuse! It's not a *time* issue. It's a *priority* issue—it's an *allocation* issue. Most Americans have plenty of time, but many of us choose to invest that time in things other than exercise.

Just for giggles, let's do some rough math regarding what we do with our time every week. See how these estimates shake out for you:

- 8 hours of sleep per day x 7 days = 56 hours
- 8 hours of work per day x 5 days = 40 hours
- 1 hour commute time per day x 5 days = 5 hours
- 2 hours of eating per day (a huge overestimation for most of us) x 7 days = 14 hours
- 1 hour grooming per day (just guessing here) x 7 days = 7 hours

That comes out to 122 hours per week. So, take 122 hours from the total 168 hours available to us (24 hours x 7 days), and that leaves 46 discretionary hours per week, or 6.57 hours per day. What are we doing with this free time? In March 2017, a company called eMarketer released its annual survey of how much time Americans spend "with media" per day. Here is the breakdown:

- Mobile (nonvoice) device: 3 hours and 23 minutes
- Desktop or laptop computer: 2 hours and 8 minutes
- Other connected devices: 30 minutes

That works out to just over six hours per day, on average. I'll admit, I'm a little leery of these numbers because they seem pretty extreme; they certainly don't align with how I spend my time, but hey, data are data. On top of this, add the national average of nearly four hours per day watching television, and it's clear many people are doing a lot of multitasking with media. It's obvious that when your eyes are glued to some sort of electronic rectangle, it's hard, if not impossible, to be physically active. Could it be that we are not moving regularly because of the magnetic power of technology? Might things like email, text messages, Facebook, Twitter, Instagram, YouTube, LinkedIn, Snapchat, Pinterest, Tinder, DVR, Netflix, Hulu, Candy Crush, and so on, consume so much of our discretionary time and mental energy that physical activity doesn't even enter the realm of possibility?

Anyone with a smartphone (which these days means *everyone*) recognizes that although the device might not control our lives and behavior, it certainly affects them. Dr. Cal Newport (who, despite the name, is not a TV weatherman in Southern California) is a professor at Georgetown University who wrote the book *Deep Work . . . Rules for Focused Success in a Distracted World*. He points out that social media is intentionally designed to distract and fragment our attention. If you don't believe Dr. Newport, honestly answer this very personal question: How long can you go without a fix? The folks at Apple claim we check our phones 80 times a day and we tap it, on average, 2,617 times a day. That is a lot of time and energy spent on your phone.

If today's inactive environment is so overwhelmingly powerful, should we all throw up our hands and declare that being healthy is simply impossible? That it's a losing proposition? *No, of course not!* We need to be two things: selfish and intentional. Being selfish means understanding that you cannot outsource your health. Of the more than seven and a half billion people on earth, no one can make healthy choices *for* you. You have to take personal responsibility and recognize that you can't pay or expect someone else to make it happen. Look in the mirror. You, and only you, hold all the power when it comes to your future and quality of life.

Being intentional means that if you have about six hours of free time per day, you are *not* going to let Mark Zuckerberg (founder of Facebook), Kevin Systrom and Mike Krieger (founders of Instagram), or Ben Silbermann (founder of Pinterest) own that time. *You* own that time! What about carving out 30 to 60 minutes daily to invest in yourself? This is not an either/or proposition. I'm certainly not advocating completely abandoning technology and social media. I'm encouraging balance. Allocate your time so that it benefits *you*, and not some venture capital-backed company in Silicon Valley that is angling for an IPO or a billion-dollar buyout.

A Special Bonus!

Because you have stuck with me this far, I have good news! You don't *always* need to invest up to 190 minutes per week in moderate-to-vigorous physical activity. If you are crunched for time, rather than just not working out at all, I suggest exploring interval training, specifically high-intensity interval training (HIIT). The concept of interval training has been around for years, but a flurry of new research really validates its benefit. Multiple studies show that by cranking up your effort (intensity), you don't have to spend as much time actually exercising. It's an inverse relationship: As your intensity goes up, your investment of time can go down. The key, though, is that you have to be willing to really push yourself (and of course be medically cleared for vigorous activity).

One of the most popular versions of HIIT is the seven-minute workout, which consists of 12 exercises you do for 30 seconds each, separated by a 10-second rest in between. The exercises need to be done at a pretty high intensity (think 8 on a scale of 1–10). You don't need to join a gym, buy expensive equipment or pay a trainer. You just need to start where you are and be consistent. It's not the *only* workout you need, but it's extremely beneficial, especially when you are traveling. For more information, Google it. You can also download a free app on your phone to help guide you through the routine (this is an example of when technology can actually *help* support physical activity). HIIT is a terrific way to keep your workouts fresh. Believe me, even though it doesn't take long, if you do it right, you will certainly *know* you've worked out.

I'll close with one of my favorite aphorisms:

> "If you don't like where you are, move.
> You are not a tree!"

"Motivation is what gets you going.
Habit is what keeps you going."
– Jim Rohn

21.

Aristotle Was Right! The Habit of Excellence

Every year in December, in addition to Christmas and Hanukkah, something amazing takes place. Across the United States, millions—yes *millions*—of Americans make their New Year's resolutions.

Harvard-trained psychologist Stephen J. Kraus has studied the science of success. He estimates that four out of every ten people make a personal commitment to do, or stop doing, something as the calendar year gets ready to turn. That "something" can include all sorts of behaviors, but more times than not, Americans' top two resolutions are to go on a diet (for weight loss) and to start exercising.

Every year, it's the same story: "Starting in January, I'm going to join a gym and lose (fill in the blank) pounds!" or "This is the year. I'm going to exercise (fill in the blank) times a week." Then what happens? One of two things: Either nothing or, if we do start exercise or weight-loss programs, we soon stop. I'm convinced that if it weren't for the month of January, the health-club industry would cease to exist. According to the research, somewhere between 88 percent and 95 percent of those who make New Year's resolutions fail to accomplish their goals.

Why are the stats so bleak? As someone immersed in the health and fitness world, I wrestle with this question regularly. Why do we do or not do what we do or don't do? I know that sounds strange. Reread that sentence slowly.

Why are some individuals amazingly successful at changing negative, unhealthy behaviors and improving their health while the majority continue to struggle for years? It turns out that humans are really complicated and changing behavior is extremely difficult. One thing is for sure: Every single one of us is incredibly unique, and why we behave the way we do is often impossible to explain.

All of the experts will tell you that your health is about 20 to 30 percent genetic (inherited from your biological mom and dad) and 70 to 80 percent a function of habits and environment (lifestyle). Obviously, you can't change your parents, but if you blame genetics for the reason you are the way you are, you're simply ignoring the facts. The vast majority of your health outcomes are up to you, no one else! Your habits—the things you do (or don't do) day in and day out—have a huge effect on your overall health. The Greek philosopher Aristotle said, "We are what we repeatedly do. Excellence, then, is not an act but a habit." That's so true! We are creatures of habit, and if we can develop healthy habits, the odds are terrific that we will improve our health.

So, here's the million-dollar question: How do you improve the odds of successfully embracing healthy habits that you can maintain for the rest of your life? How do you change *for good*?

Change Is Hard!

I've read or listened to many of the experts on behavioral change, including James Prochaska and Carlo DiClemente (the "stages of change" model), Alan Deutschman (*Change or Die*), Daniel Pink (*Drive: The Surprising Truth About What Motivates Us*), Kerry Patterson et al. (*Change Anything: The New Science of Personal Success*), Brian Wansink (*Mindless Eating: Why We Eat More Than We Think*), Charles Duhigg (*The Power of Habit: Why We Do What We Do in Life and Business*), Roy Baumeister and John Tierney (*Willpower: Rediscovering the Greatest Human Strength*), and B. J. Fogg (the behavior model). There are a multitude of theories and approaches on human behavior and change, but there seems to be one underlying point that all the experts agree on: Willpower does not work, at least not in the long run. Permanent, lasting change is not about *will*; rather, it seems to boil down to *skill*.

This is an incredibly important concept. Although you have tried in the past to make healthy lifestyle changes and have not been successful—maybe many times—that does not mean that *you* failed. It simply means that your approach or your plan failed! This is not a problem. Sharpen your skills by aggressively addressing what will increase your odds of success. Focus on *skill power* rather than *willpower*. Adjust your approach and try again. In football terms, read and react. What works for me is most likely not going to work for you. As I have told my kids for years, you learn much more from failure than from success. Understand that change is a process. Very rarely does someone flip a switch and completely change his or her behavior overnight. Be patient—the results will be worth it! The direction you are headed in is much more important than your velocity (your speed in getting to goal).

The PhDs at VitalSmarts in Provo, Utah—who do corporate training and leadership development—have authored several outstanding best-selling books, among them *Crucial Conversations: Tools for Talking When Stakes Are High*; *Crucial Accountability: Tools for Resolving Violated Expectations, Broken Commitments, and Bad Behavior*; and *Influencer: The New Science of Leading Change*. These folks talk about the importance of being both the subject and the scientist in your own experiment. Most likely, no one has ever studied *you* before. *Now* would be a great time to start. You are unique in just about every way imaginable. From your past experience, family history (DNA), occupation, religion, skill set, and schedule, to your food preferences and social networks, you name it: You are different than *everyone else* on the planet! As a result, your plan for making lifestyle changes must be structured in a way that will increase your odds of being successful. Don't expect that what your spouse/sibling/neighbor/colleague/friend/mechanic/hairdresser/cable guy tried is automatically going to work for you.

Take a step back and develop a game plan that addresses and leverages your individuality.

Now, this doesn't mean you must start from scratch. There is great credence in the adage "success leaves clues." Improving your health means changing your behavior, and because your behavior is so unique, your *plan* must be unique as well. No one is more qualified to build your plan than you are. If you try something that doesn't work, don't beat yourself up! As the VitalSmarts folks would say, "Turn a bad day into good data." Through trial and error, determine what works and what doesn't work, then adjust your plan and move forward. The more data you can collect on yourself, the greater the likelihood you will find a formula that will lead you toward success.

The Components of Behavior

B. J. Fogg believes that three things must be present for any behavior to take place: motivation, ability, and a trigger (easy to remember: B = MAT, or Behavior = Motivation + Ability + Trigger). If one of these elements is missing, behavior will simply not happen. For example, let's think about your cell phone. When your phone rings, that is the *trigger* (or call to action). If you're in a meeting or in the shower and your phone rings, you don't have the *ability* at that particular moment to answer it. If you are free to answer the call, but look at the caller ID and determine you don't want to talk to that particular person, you are lacking *motivation,* so you don't take the call. Fogg contends that all three components must be present for a new behavior to take place. Alternatively, if you want to *stop* a current behavior—smoking, eating junk food, or watching too much TV—you need to eliminate at least one of the three elements in the formula.

The fact that you are even reading this right book indicates that you have some level of motivation to improve your health. Keep in mind that motivation vacillates, so finding sources that can keep you motivated is important and is something you need to consciously address. (We will talk about the importance of your social environment in a moment.) A big question you also must answer is whether you have the *ability* to make a healthy decision. Do you have the knowledge at hand? I suggest possibly spending time with a registered dietitian and/or personal trainer to learn the basics of nutrition and exercise. You might also explore Naturally Slim, ACAP Health's weight and metabolic syndrome intervention that focuses on skill building (www.naturallyslim.com).

Creating new (healthy) habits almost *always* requires learning new skills. Once you are armed with the basics, you'll have the ability and the confidence to waltz into a restaurant, a party, a gym, etc., and easily make decisions that align with your goals (It's amazing to see the transition that takes place in a someone once that person has learned the basics). Because you were *motivated* and took the time to learn new skills, you now have the *ability* to be successful, whereas before you were just throwing darts in the dark.

Be realistic and start where you are, not where you were ten years ago or where you think you should be. Even if you were "all-state" in high school, that was probably a long time ago. Ask yourself if you have the skills necessary to develop a new behavior and, if not, what you need to do to get there. Remember, just relying on willpower will not cut it. If you are serious about embracing fitness and a healthier you, first build a strategy and then refine that strategy as you make progress. Health is a journey, not a destination.

Thelma and Louise

Health status, both good and bad, is contagious. A huge indicator of your own health is that of your social circle. Take a look at those around you—your family members, friends, and coworkers. Are they helping or hindering you in getting where you want to go? Good health is a team sport, so it's imperative to have a support network. According to data from the National Institutes of Health, you are 37 percent more likely to be obese if your spouse is obese; however, you are 171 percent more likely to become obese if your friends are obese. Do not discount the influence of those you regularly interact with. (See the upcoming chapter, "Birds of a Feather," for more on this.)

There's a possibility that the new behavior you are hoping to embrace (whether it's the habit of daily exercise, healthier eating, or quitting smoking, etc.), will make those close to you uncomfortable. If individuals in your social circle aren't interested in joining the cause of improving your health, they may actively try to derail you. These people are known as saboteurs. They may interpret your goal as a threat to their own unhealthy choices and lifestyle. That's just human nature, so don't be surprised if it happens. Be prepared to have a heart-to-heart conversation in which you actually ask for their support. They don't need to commit to do what you are doing, although that would be terrific. Simply request that they at least be supportive of your efforts. That might involve a change in what they are accustomed to in your relationship (for example, no more Thursday-night happy hours with coworkers or extra-large buttered popcorn at the movies with friends). Change is hard for everyone, not just for you. Explain to your friends and family that this goal is very important to you and that you would greatly appreciate their encouragement.

Do you remember the 1991 movie *Thelma & Louise*? Those two ladies were *very* supportive of one another. If you remember the closing scene where they drive off a cliff together, you might argue that the friendship was a tad *too* supportive. Finding someone who will support your goals will greatly increase your odds of success. Ideally, this person may even want to join you, but if not, having that person just be your cheerleader along the journey will be incredibly valuable. Make sure you let this ally know how much you appreciate the role he or she is playing in your self-improvement quest.

Again, motivation tends to ebb and flow, so surrounding yourself with the right people and tools (e.g. motivational tapes, exercise or nutrition classes, inspirational books, and athletic events) will immensely increase your odds of success. Other "fuel for your fire" might be watching or volunteering at a race like a 5K, 10K, marathon, or triathlon; just being in that healthy, positive environment can motivate you to improve your health and fitness. Cheering for the participants along race routes and at the finish lines can be very inspiring!

What about Your Environment?

As president of a health-consulting firm, I work in an incredibly healthy environment. I'm surrounded by a group of health-conscience colleagues with an equipment-laden gym in my office building, and my membership to that fitness center is free. Just outside of my building is a twenty-plus-mile trail perfect for walking, running, or cycling. My close friends include board-certified physicians, PhDs, registered dietitians, exercise physiologists, nurses, and personal trainers. If I have a question or problem regarding my own health and fitness goals, I can pick up the phone or send an e-mail and have an answer within minutes. At home, I have easy access to beautiful enormous parks that include soccer and baseball fields, basketball courts, and running and cycling trails that are part of a citywide system. I have a son who loves to work out and a dog that wants multiple walks a day. I am also a member of the local YMCA, which is close enough to walk to if I choose. As you might imagine, I don't have a lot of excuses regarding exercise, especially as it relates to my environment. I realize I'm blessed to live in such an awesome community, but I didn't end up here by accident. Dr. David Katz at Yale says, "The choices we make are a function of the choices we have." Knowing this, my wife Kathy and I were very intentional about choosing where to live when we moved from Arizona to Texas when our kids were young.

What about *your* environment? Studies show that a supportive environment plays a giant role in your ability to be healthy. A

2010 paper published by WELCOA (the Wellness Council of America) focused on the factors influencing behavior change. The number-one factor, accounting for 40 percent of the effect on behavior change, was "opportunity," of which environment is a major component. "Readiness" accounted for 30 percent, "skill" was 25 percent, and "awareness" 5 percent. The odds are high that your environment, both at work and at home, is either helping or hurting your embrace of a healthy lifestyle. Take an inventory of your environment and see how you might modify any of the road-blocks or speed bumps. Realistically assess how your immediate world is affecting your behavior, positively or negatively.

If you are thinking of a workout location or considering join-ing a gym, be sure to make it convenient to your current routine. If you have to make a big effort to get there, you will significantly reduce the odds of it ever becoming a regular part of your routine; the more effort or thought required for a behavior, the less likely it's going to happen. Consider your current daily schedule. The things you do *without thinking* are the things you do on a regular basis (i.e., your habits): brushing your teeth, taking your vitamins, putting on your seatbelt, and so on.

There is a big difference between "compliance" and "habit." You need to be mindful of your plan for achieving your goals and desired behavior. Individuals can do just about anything for a short time (compliance), but for a behavior to truly become a part of your regular routine (habit), you need to consciously reduce the barriers to entry. Selecting a location to exercise outside of your usual travel pattern is a plan that's almost guaranteed to eventually fail.

Triggers and the Use of Technology

Technology has played a significant role in contributing to many of the country's public-health problems, including obesity, inactivity, diabetes, loneliness and depression. Physical activity has basically become optional for most Americans, including our children. A 2016 study by Statista found that children between 12 and 17 spent more than 21 hours per week playing video games, smartphone surfing and/or watching TV. The weekly multimedia allotment for kids 2 to 11 years old was more than 26 and a half hours! The good news is, I'm convinced we can also use technology to help us get up and off the couch.

We talked earlier about the importance of triggers, an integral component of any behavior (along with ability and motivation). Cell phones, especially smartphones, can serve as excellent triggers. You can program your phone to send you e-mails and texts, even to sound alarms. This is the modern-day version of tying a string around your finger to remind you to do something important (like exercise!). Remember that you must have a trigger to initiate whatever you are hoping to do, so take advantage of technology. It can be a tremendous ally.

You might make technology your friend by using a wearable, a device worn on the body that automatically tracks activity (such as steps per day) and, often, sleep and heart rate. Loads of cool software available on the market (much of it can be downloaded free to your laptop or smartphone) can log your daily food and drink intake, as well as your physical activity. These devices can even be programmed to vibrate to remind you to break up bouts of sedentary behavior during your workday.

This "accelerometer space" in the marketplace is crowded and changes almost monthly. Some of the most popular devices include Fitbit, Nike Fuel Band, Garmin's VivoFit, and others. They can be worn on your wrist, waist, or shoe, and even as jewelry. Remember that none of the wearables are exact, but they do give you a good indication of how you are tracking. In other words, they help you be mindful.

Dr. Fogg believes that the best way to ensure success is to "put hot triggers in front of motivated people." A hot trigger is something you can act on *right now*, like an alarm clock or a red traffic light turning green, as opposed to a cold trigger (which you can't act on immediately, such as a billboard advertising a local gym membership). In Dallas, where I live, it gets pretty hot in the summer. I often have to water the trees and plants in our yard to keep them from burning up. I used to turn on the water, come inside, and inevitably get busy doing something else. By the time I remembered that the water was still on, it was often too late. The ground had become saturated and the water would be flowing into the street. The solution? Simple...my smartphone! I estimate how long the water needs to be on, set the alarm, and go about my business. When the alarm goes off, it reminds me, "Hey, dummy, don't forget the water." Works every time!

The point is that initially, I kept trying to remember on my own, to use willpower to help me accomplish the task ("I'll just *really* concentrate this time and I won't forget!"). What I actually needed was to take a step back, determine a fresh strategy, and try again. I encourage you to do the same with whatever your goals are. Leveraging technology, in particular on your smartphone, might give you the edge you need. Wearing an activity tracker and using it along with a smartphone app like MyFitnessPal will potentially help you initiate the habit of regular physical activity.

The Importance of Baby Steps

You'll recall from earlier chapters that the research is overwhelming that if you want to receive the phenomenal benefits of exercise, you need 150 minutes of moderate physical activity per week, and that you can cut that time in half if you increase the intensity from moderate to vigorous. Because there are 168 hours in a week, from my perspective, 150 minutes (less than three hours!) doesn't seem like much—but published studies using accelerometer data indicate no more than 25 percent of American adults reach the 150-minute target.

I have come to the conclusion that *my perspective* is not what's important if I want to help people get active. I'm already a regular exerciser. Exercise is a habit for me; it's what I do, who I am. To me, the 150-minute target, or 30 minutes per day most days of the week, doesn't seem like much. I'm already there. In "stages of change" terminology, I am in the maintenance phase. For someone *thinking* about starting an exercise program (e.g., in the contemplation phase), however, half an hour of exercise a day can seem like an insurmountable task. I might as well be asking that person to train for a marathon or an Ironman triathlon (2.4-mile swim, 112-mile bike ride, and 26-mile run—yikes!). Asking someone to go from zero activity to thirty minutes a day doesn't make sense, at least from a behavior-modification standpoint. Mentally, it's often too large of a hurdle.

What *does* make sense is to ask someone to take a baby step. How about walking *three* minutes a day? That's it, just three minutes! You can walk inside, outside, or in place. Just commit to doing that every day for five days. You might be thinking that three minutes will not offer any significant health benefit, and you would be absolutely right—but that's not the point. Just getting into the habit or routine of regular physical activity is critical to ultimately move up to the prescribed dose of 150 minutes a week.

A great example of the importance of baby steps is Dr. Fogg's recommendation to "floss one tooth." The oral hygiene experts will tell you that regularly flossing your teeth is at least as important, if not more important, than brushing your teeth. Most of us have been told by our dentists or dental hygienists to floss daily. However, when I ask large audiences to raise their hands if they floss regularly, usually only about 50–60 percent raise their hands.

Why is that? If we know it's good for us, why don't we do it? We most likely have been taught to floss, so we obviously have the ability. Flossing doesn't take long. It's not expensive. And it's very beneficial. The fact that flossing can improve our health and substantially lower our risk of gum disease and infection should offer plenty of motivation, yet many of us still don't floss. Could it be that if you're a non-flosser, flossing all your teeth will hurt, maybe for a couple days, and your gums will most likely bleed, maybe a lot? If you're not used to it, the "sharp" floss will be painful. That makes total sense! For cryin' out loud, we're human and we don't like to hurt! We know that the pain will not last forever, but that is irrelevant. It's hard for the long-term benefits to outweigh the short-term painful speed bumps. How can we get over that? What about deciding that once a day, right after brushing your teeth, you are going to floss "just one tooth"? Just one, no more. If you bleed at all, it won't be much, and if it's painful, the pain will be minimal.

The goal is to take something that is already a habit (brushing your teeth) and "bolt on" a new behavior immediately following that activity. The brushing of the teeth serves as the trigger, and once you have "trained the cycle" of "brush-floss, brush-floss," before long, those two separate behaviors become one. Suddenly, you become a consistent flosser without having to think about it. Obviously, after a while, you will naturally start expanding the behavior from one tooth to three or four, and then to *all* of your teeth.

So, remember, there is a big difference between *knowing* and *doing*. Having the knowledge that a behavior is beneficial will have zero impact until you are able to actually *do* the behavior consistently. You may think that using baby steps is too simplistic, but I challenge you to think about your past success rate. How has just relying on willpower worked for you? If you can start gradually and train the cycle by removing the perceived barriers, before you know it, you will have developed a healthy habit. I encourage you to try this method with walking, flossing, or adding fruits or vegetables to your daily intake.

Healthy habits are contagious, and *your* health is *your* responsibility. Select a realistic goal that's important to you, then build a plan, enlist a support network, and start with baby steps. Soon, you'll be well on your way to a healthy lifestyle. You'll most likely feel better, look better, sleep better, and have fewer aches and pains, more energy, and more confidence! Aristotle was right…small changes can provide amazing results. Habits are the key!

"A year from now you will wish you had started today."

"You drown not by falling into a river,
but by staying submerged in it."
– Paulo Cuelho

22.

Everybody Has Stuff:
Speed Bumps, Roadblocks, and Detours

Because I'm a health and wellness guy and speak to various groups around the country, I often meet folks who have recently radically improved their health—men and women who in the past year or two have completely reversed course on the direction they were headed. They've lost weight, started eating nutritious and satisfying food, embraced regular physical activity, been able to go off many of their meds, and dramatically improved their energy and outlook. I love meeting these people! They are health evangelists and want desperately to share their message. They'd like everyone to reap the rewards they now understand are available to us all.

Whenever possible, I take a few minutes and ask such people these questions: What triggered the change? What was it that made you decide that the status quo was not working? Why were you suddenly motivated to invest in yourself?

"Why?" is a question I'm constantly trying to answer. I believe the answer to that question is the Holy Grail. If I could find it, I'd be able to help millions of people enjoy wonderful, healthy lives. I know it can be done. I see and hear about it regularly. I used to believe that success was simply knowing right from wrong (i.e., when you know better, you do better), but I have learned that is clearly not the case! I can stop one hundred people at any mall in America and ask, "Is smoking bad for your health?" A full 100 percent will say, "Yes!" I'd get the same consensus if I were to ask if exercising or if eating fruits and vegetables provides benefits, although fifty years ago, that would not have been the case. Today, most people pretty much know right from wrong, at least in terms of basic behaviors that influence health.

Even though I don't have iron-clad data to support it, I believe that the real issue keeping people from improving their health is their "stuff." Everybody has stuff—the issues that get in our way, the things that prevent us from being successful. These speed bumps, roadblocks, and detours live between our ears. Our stuff, real or imagined, can be very powerful, leading to all sorts of excuses.

What's your stuff? What's holding you back? What's keeping you from having a healthy, happy, productive life? What's your excuse? This can be a very difficult question to answer. Being truly honest with yourself can be pretty uncomfortable.

Experience has taught me that for many people's stuff stems from something that happened a long time ago, often in childhood. It may be something as simple as a single comment from a teacher, friend, spouse, or, often, parent. If that's the source of your stuff, ask yourself, "How is that view, perspective, or comment *helping* me now? And *why* am I letting it affect me?"

One Woman's Story

A few years back, I had a conversation with a former coworker, Deb, at the Cooper Aerobics Center. I'd known Deb professionally for more than twelve years. She is a PowerPoint goddess and often helped me add sizzle to my presentations. When I sat down in her office, she leaned over, looked me in the eye, lowered her voice, and whispered, "I've lost twenty-six pounds."

I said, "Wow, congratulations! Since when?"

Over the previous five months, she told me. Deb had worked at Cooper for nineteen years. She had daily direct contact with Dr. Ken Cooper, commonly known as the father of aerobics, and full access to a world-class fitness center, personal trainers, and dietitians.

The campus is an epicenter of health and preventive medicine. Despite access to all of that, Deb had struggled with her weight and fitness. (By the way, I'm not talking out of school; Deb graciously agreed to let me share her story.) So why now? What triggered the change? Deb's response was incredibly moving.

As it turns out, Deb's only child, Ashley, who lives in New York, had recently had a baby. Ashley had grown up in Dallas and always had a wonderful relationship with her mom and dad. After high school, she had gone to college in New York. Though Deb missed her daughter very much, she totally supported Ashley's decision. In the back of her mind, Deb always thought that Ashley would return home to Texas after she graduated. Well, Ashley really liked the Northeast, and after completing college, she had stayed there, taking a job in New York. Even though Deb never let on, she shared with me that she had been devastated by Ashley's decision. With tears in her eyes, Deb realized that her only child had a new home, and it wasn't just around the corner—it was halfway across the country!

This devastation had become Deb's stuff. She harbored a terribly empty feeling that was ever present, but, not wanting to put her daughter on a guilt trip, Deb just "kept pushing it down." For whatever reason, she felt that the best way for her to deal with these feelings was *not* to deal with them. When Ashley got married in 2010, the reality was magnified yet again, but Deb never communicated her feelings. She continued to suppress them, and as she did, her weight went up and her health went down.

Ashley then had a baby boy, Yoon-Mo, and of course the proud grandparents went to New York to meet their new grandbaby. As you might expect, Deb believed her grandson was the most beautiful baby ever, and the visit was wonderful, yet, upon returning home, Deb found that her empty feelings were as strong as ever. She finally decided she needed some help. She scheduled an appointment with a therapist, Dr. Pam Walker, whom she had known for years.

Initially, Deb's conversations with Dr. Walker focused on Deb's feelings, her internalized anger, and why she was so stuck.

After the first month, Dr. Walker asked Deb if she was getting any exercise. Deb said no, that really, she just shut down every day after work and took solace in her Blue Bell ice cream (for you non-Texans, Blue Bell is a regional brand that has magical qualities!). Dr. Walker made Deb promise to cut out the ice cream for four months and encouraged her to try to walk every day, to get some sunlight. This was outstanding advice, as research shows that both exercise and vitamin D (either from the sun or from supplements) can improve both mood and life satisfaction.

Dr. Walker discovered something else during therapy: Deb hadn't had a physical or a blood profile done in more than six years. Remember, Deb worked at a facility that is recognized as one of the world's leading preventive medicine clinics. She knew as well as anyone how important a regular physical exam was, especially for anyone older than forty, but she was scared. She believed she had probably developed diabetes, and she didn't want to know it. Her *stuff* had taken control of her health and her life!

As it turned out, even though Deb's blood work was not ideal, she was not diabetic and she was in much better shape than she had imagined. She felt as if a rock had been lifted.

Dr. Walker continued to help Deb understand her feelings and gave her the opportunity to share what had been tying her up in knots for almost ten years. The process was cathartic, and as Deb began to *think* better, she began to *act* better. She became more mindful of her eating and of her physical activity, and she started losing weight and feeling better—much better!

Deb's daughter, son-in-law, and grandbaby, Yoon-Mo, came for a visit, and after dinner one night, Deb shared with Ashley what had been going on with her. She told Ashley that she was seeing a therapist and how she was working through many of the issues that had become such a burden. Now, handling her stuff, Deb felt so much better. Incredibly supportive, Ashley is thrilled that her mom is doing so well.

Deb had lost weight, but, much more important, she *felt* 1,000 percent better! She knows, looking forward, that the quantity and quality of time she will be able to spend with her beautiful grandson will be tremendously enhanced.

Dealing with Stuff

Everybody has stuff. The question is, how are you going to deal with yours? It's not *what* happens to you that's important; it's how you *handle* what happens to you. *You* are in charge of that; no one else is. Think about what might be keeping you from embracing a healthier lifestyle. Quit making excuses, and quit trying to fool yourself. If you want to get better, you can—and you will!

For years, I have told my kids, "Your priorities are defined by what you do, not by what you say." Start *doing* the right things, and the results will be phenomenal. It all starts between the ears, but there is a huge difference between *knowing* and *doing*. Get a handle on your stuff. Get some help from someone if need be: a therapist, friend, minister, rabbi, or your doctor. You are not the Lone Ranger! Let go of whatever is holding you back, and start enjoying all the benefits that come with improved health! The return on your investment will be monumental!

"Don't let mental blocks control you.
Set yourself free.
Confront your fear and turn the mental blocks
into building blocks."
- Rooplean

Sage Advice

In the late 1990s, I had the honor of interviewing the great Dr. Stephen Covey, best known for his international bestseller, *The 7 Habits of Highly Effective People*. We actually spent most of our time discussing his latest book, *The 7 Habits of Highly Effective Families*, and he shared an incredibly important lesson that I've applied throughout my life.

Dr. Covey had nine children and, as he told me, "28 and-a-half grandchildren." (When he passed away in 2012, he had 52 grandkids.) My own kids were eight and 10 at the time, and I asked Dr. Covey, "If you had just one piece of advice for a young father, what would it be?"

I can still hear his response, delivered in his deep, thoughtful manner. "I'll share the Asian motto," he told me. "When you bow, bow low." He went on to elaborate that as a parent, you are bound to make mistakes—we all do; when it happens, say, "I'm sorry. I made a mistake. I shouldn't have done that." And then stop. Never apologize with a caveat. In other words, don't say, "I'm sorry, *but* the only reason I did what I did is because you (fill in the blank)." When you bow, bow low.

Turns out, I've found this lesson is important for me to use with not only my children, but all of the people in my life, including my wife, Kathy, my friends, colleagues, business associates and even strangers. Often, what we call an apology is just a thinly veiled justification for our regrettable behavior. If you simply and sincerely say, "I'm sorry," it often can remove a great deal of the stuff that may be influencing your life and your relationships.

*"You'll never leave where you are
until you decide where you'd rather be."*

23.

Birds of a Feather: Who's on Your Team?

Peer-reviewed studies on health and fitness can be quite thought-provoking. A perfect example was an article published in the December 2012 issue of the *Journal of Social and Personal Relationships* about "mixed-weight couples," in which one partner is overweight and the other isn't. Researchers from the University of Puget Sound and the University of Arizona studied forty-three heterosexual couples and found those in the "mixed-weight" category experienced more relationship conflict, including resentfulness and anger, than so-called same-weight couples. Results indicated that those couples with the most conflict involved a healthy-weight man and an overweight woman. When just the man was overweight, interestingly, there wasn't much conflict.

It's not news that men and women are different. John Gray made that very clear in his 1993 best-selling book *Men Are from Mars, Women Are from Venus: The Classic Guide to Understanding the Opposite Sex.* Weight is a touchy subject, and when it comes to relationships, one should always tread lightly; however, while "mixed-weight" couples certainly exist, they are not the norm. We know that those people in our support network, including spouses, have a huge influence on our behaviors and habits and, ultimately, our weight. A study published in the July 2007 issue of the *New England Journal of Medicine* found that if your spouse is obese, you are 37 percent more likely to be obese. You might be surprised to learn that if your friends are obese, you are 171 percent more likely to be obese. As I often say, when it comes to your health, which includes your weight, you are not the Lone Ranger.

Problems can arise when a significant other starts a self-improvement program that might include an increase in physical activity and a healthy-eating *kick* (a term that always makes me smile). It's common for the recent convert to want his or her partner to join in this new healthy way of living. If this describes you, I caution you to walk before you run. Remember the adage "When the student is ready, the teacher will appear." Only when the *student* is *ready*. It's human nature that once you participate in a positive experience, you want to share it with those you love. The problem, however, is if your loved one isn't *ready* to change, your unbridled enthusiasm will most likely not be received as you intend it. In fact, it might completely backfire, which could potentially extinguish *your* flame. I'm not saying this always happens . . . just don't be surprised if it does.

Change is difficult, and when a spouse or close friend decides to change, even if it's a positive change, it can often be viewed as a threat to the one being "left behind." Questions like these could be raised: "What's wrong with the way we've been living/eating/exercising all these years? Am I suddenly not good enough for you?" Change on the part of one partner can lead to some difficult, but necessary, conversations. Dr. Fogg teaches that as humans, we are lazy, social, and creatures of habit. Having allies can be phenomenally helpful, but we are all unique, and when it comes to change, those we love don't always move at the same speed as others.

If this is the case in your relationship, here's a script you might want to share with your loved one: "As you know, I'm pretty excited about my new commitment to improve my health. I also know that you're not really on board with all the changes. I get that. I'd love for you to join me in my journey, but if you're not interested, that's okay. I will still love you and hope you will continue to love me too. All I ask is that you support me and try not to derail me. My *new* routine may mean that some of our *old* routine may be affected. I'll do what I can to minimize that, but please try to be my cheerleader. Your support will be a huge part of my success. Are you okay with that?"

Then just listen. This may be a tense conversation, but it will be far easier if it happens early in your journey rather than after tension and conflict have become major issues in the relationship. Recruiting a teammate, or teammates, can be critical to your long-term success. You will definitely need to avoid Debbie Downer—the "friend" who does everything she or he can to constantly challenge why you would be interested in getting better/healthier/stronger. A focused conversation with Debbie may be necessary, but I suggest no more than two of these talks. If Debbie doesn't get it, you may need to curtail your interaction with her.

The research indicates that the "birds of a feather" theory is more common than "opposites attract." If all or most of your friends smoke, odds are, you smoke. If all or most of your friends ride bikes, I bet you do as well. Improving your health and building beneficial habits requires intention. Part of that process is evaluating if those around you are helping or hurting your cause. Remember, for long term success, your community matters—a lot!

"If you keep doing what you've been doing,
you'll keep getting what you've been getting."
– Zig Ziglar

"If it's important to you, you will find a way.
If it's not, you'll find an excuse."

24.

Sleep: The Third Leg of the Stool

When it comes to health, many of us focus primarily on two things: diet and exercise. We've heard it for years, the same mantra over and over—diet and exercise, diet and exercise—from doctors, octogenarians, personal trainers, Oprah, you name it. The prescription is always the same. While I'll be the first to admit that diet and exercise are critical components of a healthy, rewarding life, they don't provide 100 percent of the return on investment. There is another vitally important factor: sleep.

How much sleep did *you* get last night? The experts tell us that adults need seven to nine hours per night. Infants, children, and teenagers need more than that. The National Sleep Foundation has a terrific chart on how much sleep is recommended per age group (http://sleepfoundation.org/how-sleep-works/how-much-sleep-do-we-really-need). Is everyone getting the recommended amount in your house? Probably not. The truth is that millions of Americans struggle to get through the day because of problems they have getting through the night. There's a reason that Starbucks and Dunkin' Donuts do killer business and that men, women, and even *children* routinely drop three dollars or more daily for so-called energy shots or drinks.

Are You a "Short Sleeper"?

A short sleeper is defined as someone who gets fewer than six hours of sleep per night and still functions normally throughout the day. Sleep patterns typically begin in childhood or adolescence and sustain into adulthood. Researchers believe sleep patterns might stem from gene mutations. It's estimated that just one percent of American adults are true short sleepers.

So, what about the 99 percent of the rest of us? Studies indicate around 40 percent of American adults average less than seven hours of sleep per night. And that's a problem. Most of us can reasonably manage after an occasional restless night, but continual lack of adequate sleep has a cumulative effect. Over time, lack of sleep can really take a toll. Research shows that two weeks of sleeping only six hours a night has the same effect of one or two nights of complete sleep deprivation.

Studies also indicate that lost and low-quality sleep increase "cyberloafing," which is when employees spend time surfing the net while on the clock (this according to an article by David T. Wagner et al. in the September 2012 issue of the *Journal of Applied Psychology*). What does this lack of productivity cost an organization? Plenty! There are other, more serious risks with sleep deprivation, too. The Centers for Disease Control estimate that between 15 and 33 percent of all fatal car crashes involve a driver who did not get adequate sleep.

Is Technology to Blame?

Technology is powerful. If you're under thirty, you take technology for granted, but any baby boomer will tell you that the world we live in today is radically different than "when we grew up." Cell phones have become ubiquitous, and of course cell phones are rarely used to make phone calls. They are really just hyper-functional, at-the-ready mobile computers. Everyone—and I mean *everyone*—now has a smartphone (okay, maybe not that one guy at the office that loves to exhibit his 2001 flip phone with the worn-out 3, but he's a dinosaur).

The things that smartphones allow us to do are amazing: check and respond to e-mail, surf the Internet, get directions, shoot HD photos and video, listen to music, watch movies and TV shows, play games, and connect with friends and strangers all over the world through text, voice, and video. That little rectangular device you keep in your purse or pocket is magnetic. We can't avoid checking our phones multiple times per day—at work, while standing in line at the bank or grocery store, while eating, just about *everywhere*. Look around at any restaurant. You'll see couples staring at their phones, not saying a word to one another, and families, every single member silently mesmerized by something on his or her screen. Parents' phones have become the go-to distraction for antsy toddlers—children who can't even speak yet entranced for hours, looking at pictures or playing games on small screens. Dr. Gary Small, in his book *iBrain: Surviving the Technological Alteration of the Modern Mind*, states that "perhaps not since Early Man discovered how to use a tool has the human brain been affected so quickly and dramatically."

So, what's my point? Technology is addicting, and not by accident. There are tens of thousands of *really* smart people—PhD smart—working right now to get you to do what they want. The reason the folks at Facebook created the ability to tag someone in a photo is to influence behavior. Their business model is based on getting people to their website . . . and keeping them there. That's the definition of their business. It's how they make money, and it's working really well!

How does this all tie in to sleep? Simple. The temptation to keep playing Angry Birds, Words with Friends, Candy Crush, or Grand Theft Auto effectively overrides our biological need for sleep—even at night, when we are sleepy! Without even really weighing the pros and cons, we opt for "just one more game" before bed. Or we move from one text to a tweet that links us to an article that includes an embedded video of a waterskiing squirrel or a baby that can't stop giggling.

And it's not just smartphones, tablets, and laptops that command our attention. The DVR is an equally powerful tool. We can record multiple episodes of the same television show and become binge viewers, watching consecutive episodes of weekly programs during a single sitting. A commercial-free hour of *Breaking Bad* (or *This Is Us, Orange Is the New Black, Game of Thrones, Homeland, The Walking Dead, Sons of Anarchy, Arrow*—whatever your show of choice) is awesome! Sure, it's 11:15 p.m., and you should probably go to bed, but just one more episode . . . Don't think for a minute that the writers and producers of those shows don't use every trick they can to get you to come back for more. That's their business! It's no different than the big food companies leveraging neuroscience to formulate "foods" that are cheap, convenient, and great-tasting. Whether the company is selling you "food" or entertainment, the goal is to manipulate your behavior to benefit their bottom line. Reed Hastings, the CEO of Netflix, once claimed that the three biggest competitors to his digital movie and TV programming platform were Facebook, YouTube and sleep.

How Much Is Enough?

The first step in correcting the problem is assessing if you currently get enough sleep. Remember, adults should be targeting seven to nine hours per night. If you are among the millions of Americans who should be getting more sleep, it helps to know about sleep hygiene. The National Sleep Foundation defines "sleep hygiene" as a variety of practices that are necessary for people to have normal, quality nighttime sleep and full daytime alertness. The most important element in improving the quality and quantity of sleep appears to be establishing a consistent routine. Going to bed and getting up at close to the same times every day, even on weekends, is critical for producing appropriate sleep. There is tremendous individual variability when it comes to sleep, so consider these suggestions as food for thought:

- *Avoid or limit caffeine if you happen to be caffeine sensitive.* My good friend Dr. Craig Schwimmer, a Dallas-based ear-nose-and-throat doctor, recommends cutting off all coffee, tea, caffeine-laden soft drinks, and chocolate (sorry!) after 1:00 p.m. if you are having challenges with sleep at night. Nicotine is a stimulant, so also knock that off (eliminating this would obviously also provide a plethora of other health and economic benefits).

- *Limit or avoid alcohol.* Alcohol can often promote *getting* to sleep, but it can cause problems *staying* asleep once the body starts metabolizing it.

- *Cool down your environment.* When it comes to room temperature for sleep, cooler seems to be better. Most studies indicate that a room temperature between 60 and 67 degrees Fahrenheit is optimal for sleeping, with temperatures above 75 degrees and below 54 degrees disruptive to sleep. Body temperature has also been linked to the amount of deep sleep you're able to get, with cooler body temperatures promoting more deep sleep.

- *Darken the bedroom.* Create a dark environment in your bedroom that restricts or limits outside light. Alarm clock screens, nightlights, and exposure to outside floodlights can be disruptive to sleep.

- *Limit activity in bed.* Watching TV, reading (especially on a screen), or writing in bed, for most people, negatively affects sleep patterns. Again, this varies from person to person.

- *Give yourself appropriate wind-down time.* Avoid watching television shows that promote extreme emotions for at least an hour before heading to the bedroom. Watching an episode of *C.S.I.* or *The Blacklist* right before bed is not a great idea. This obviously applies to video games as well. Start winding down at least an hour before you try to go to sleep.

- *Take a hot shower or bath.* For some, taking a hot shower or bath right before sliding under cool sheets in a quiet, dark bedroom seems to work great. The shower or bath raises the core body temperature, but when you then accelerate the cooling process, it works to promote the transition to sleep.

- *Don't eat too close to bedtime.* Eating right before bed can not only upset your stomach, but can also throw off your ability to metabolize what you ate while you sleep.

- *Exercise regularly.* Exercise can be very helpful in promoting sleep; however, I've found there is a huge variance in how people respond to physical activity as it relates to sleep. Some, myself included, can work out hard at night, take a quick shower, and be asleep within minutes. Others find it difficult to get to sleep shortly after a workout. Overall, most of the research shows that consistent exercisers are also pretty good sleepers, so you'll need to find the best time for you to work out and still sleep.

- *Try melatonin.* Despite plenty of Internet claims that no effective sleep supplements seem to exist, one exception for many people is melatonin. There are two available versions: a quick-acting version for those who have trouble getting to sleep, and a time-release version for those who get to sleep easily but have trouble staying asleep. Generally, 1-3 milligrams per night is an appropriate dose, but don't depend on melatonin every night. Recent studies have found repeated use of melatonin will eventually blunt the supplement's ability to aid sleep.

- *Manage your technology!* All the experts will tell you that staying connected 24/7 is not healthy. Set boundaries, and don't feel compelled to answer an e-mail or text after a certain time at night. Yes, I know many people have jobs that include colleagues and customers all over the country (or world), but your overall effectiveness will be negatively affected if you don't allow yourself some downtime or "me" time. Draw a line—say 7:00 p.m.—and stick to it!

The Bottom Line

The evidence is pretty clear that lack of adequate sleep negatively affects just about every area of your life, so although diet and exercise still rank at the top of the list for improving health, don't downplay the importance of sleep. It's definitely the third leg of the stool.

> "Finish each day and be done with it.
> You have done what you could.
> Learn from it; tomorrow is a new day."
> – Ralph Waldo Emerson

"Age is a case of mind over matter.
If you don't mind, it don't matter."
– Satchel Paige

25.

Take a Seat: The Brazilian Sit-Stand Test

From a guy who normally recommends walking the dog even if you don't have one, the suggestion to take a seat seems somewhat contradictory, I know, but bear with me. A study done by researchers in Brazil and published the *European Journal of Cardiovascular Prevention* concluded that testing a person's ability to sit down on the floor and then rise can predict how long he or she will live. That's right, the less support you need to sit down on the floor and then stand back up is an outstanding predictor of your future. The researchers tested more than two thousand men and women between the ages of fifty-one and eighty. Those who needed the most support for the process of sitting down and standing up, including bracing with a knee, hand, or both, had more than six times greater risk of dying within the next six years. (Speed was not a factor in the assessment.)

When I speak to groups about the correlation between health, fitness, and longevity, I often ask them to stand up from their chairs without using their arms. This is one of the many activities of daily living that experts use to assess frailty and disability. (Other functional activities include dressing yourself, feeding yourself, using the bathroom without assistance, and walking down a hallway and back in a prescribed amount of time.) The ability to rise from a chair using leg power only is a good indicator of lower body and core strength, flexibility, and balance. These outcomes are related to the risk of falls and fractures, which are major concerns for older adults. These abilities are also directly related to quality of life. If you can't stand up without using your arms, your lifestyle is compromised and you are, by definition, limited. You can push back the onset of disability by between thirteen and twenty years by maintaining your fitness level. That's huge!

By now, I wouldn't be surprised if you have tested yourself on the Brazilian sit-stand test. Getting a perfect score of ten is the goal: five for sitting and five for standing. Points and half points are deducted for things like touching a hand or knee to the ground while sitting or pushing off with a hand on one knee on the way up. If you wobble on the way up or down, that will cost you half a point each. In the Brazilian study, more than half of the subjects between seventy-six and eighty failed the tests, scoring three points or less. A whopping 70 percent of those under sixty earned perfect or near-perfect scores of eight, nine, or ten. The higher your score, the higher your ratio of muscle power to body weight—and the longer you will live.

No matter your score, you can improve that ratio—and your overall quality of life—with activities such as weight training, yoga, Pilates, Zumba, kettlebells, and swimming. Remember, it doesn't matter where you are; what matters is the direction you are headed. The goal is to *live,* not just to *be alive.* By maintaining your fitness as you age, and by keeping up your strength and balance, you'll drastically reduce your risk of falling and breaking a hip.

> "Live your life and forget your age."
> – Norman Vincent Peale

"The benefit of Vitamin D is as clear as the harmful link between smoking and lung cancer."
– Dr. Cedrick Garland

26.

What about Supplements?

The most important thing I can tell you about nutritional supplements is that they are aptly named. They are *supplements,* but not *replacements,* for a well-balanced, healthy diet. Ideally, *all* of your nutrition— your protein, fat, and carbohydrates, along with your vitamins and minerals— should come from the food you consume. The problem is, there's a big difference between *ideal* and *real.*

We are all different, but when it comes to what we eat, we are *really* different. Just take a look what other people have in their shopping carts at the grocery store. There is enormous variety in terms of what individuals consume daily. Obviously, I can't analyze *your* individual diet here, but most Americans are lacking (some of us woefully) nutrients. Whenever you allow someone you don't know to cook what you eat (i.e., when you dine out), you have pretty much lost control of your nutrition. As discussed, restaurants, along with the huge companies that manufacture food products, are interested in primarily one thing: getting you to like/enjoy/crave their product. Unfortunately, what tastes great is not always good for us.

In this land of plenty, it might surprise you to learn that many Americans are malnourished despite being overweight or obese. When we look collectively at what Americans eat (large quantities of non-nourishing food), it's easy to understand why. So where should you start when it comes to supplements? I suggest with the low-hanging fat (pardon the pun).

Omega-3 Fatty Acids

At the very top of my list are omega-3 fatty acids, the healthiest of all fats. Omega-3 is now the number-one best-selling nutritional supplement in the world. Since 1971, more than 32,000 published studies have noted the benefits of omega-3s. We get these oils primarily from fish—not just any fish, but such "fatty, cold-water fish" as salmon, trout, mackerel, sardines, herring, and anchovies.

The story of how omega-3s were "discovered" is fascinating. In the late 1960s, two Danish researchers, Dr. Olaf Bang and Dr. Jorn Dyerberg, were curious about why Greenland's native population, the Inuit, had 90 percent lower risk for heart disease than Denmark's population (at the time, Greenland was a Danish territory). The Inuit population achieved this despite consuming seal blubber as a primary source of nutrition (it's pretty tough to grow fruits and veggies in Greenland).

The young researchers scrambled to raise funds to make the journey across the Atlantic. Once in Greenland, they took a boat to a northern port, then used sled dogs to get to a very remote, isolated area known as Igdlorssuit. Then—this is amazing—Bang and Dyerberg convinced 130 Inuits to allow them to take blood samples (that must have been an interesting negotiation). When the researchers analyzed the blood samples, they discovered two large spikes they had never seen before. Turns out, those spikes were EPA and DHA, the so-called long-chain fatty acids that we now know to be beneficial to our health. These are *essential* fats, which means our bodies can't make them and we must therefore consume them. EPA and DHA come primarily from the microalgae that fish eat. In the case of the Inuit, the fish ate the algae, the seals ate the fish, and the Inuit ate the seals. It appeared that the nutritionist Adelle Davis was right: We really *are* what we eat.

Bang and Dyerberg published their exciting discovery in the British medical journal *The Lancet* in June 1971. That's what got the ball rolling on the omega-3s. Today, we know that the omega-3s play a critical role in keeping cell membranes healthy and efficient. That's why the list of omega-3 benefits is so long. If you do a PubMed (www.pubmed.gov) search on omega-3s, you will find thousands of published studies showing that omega-3s positively affect all sorts of conditions, including cardiovascular health, fetal development, memory and cognition, mood, vision, inflammation, and aging.

The bottom line is that if you eat any of the fatty fish listed earlier at least two or more times per week, you probably don't need to take an omega-3 supplement ("omega-3" and "fish oil" are not the same, but in the marketplace, they are often used interchangeably). The challenge is that the average American eats fish only once every eleven days (by the way, fried catfish and fillet-o-fish don't count!). As a result, studies reveal that the average blood levels of EPA+ DHA, as measured by the HS-Omega-3 Index, in the United States is only about 4–5 percent. In Japan, the average is over 8 percent, which is not surprising since as a culture the Japanese often eat fish two or three times *a day*.

If I could take only one nutritional supplement a day, it would be omega-3. The key is to get at least 1,000 mg of EPA+DHA (combined) per day. You can certainly take more if you'd like; the Inuits averaged about 14,000 mg per day! If you happen to have high triglycerides, the research indicates that you will need to take at least 3,000 mg of EPA+DHA combined per day. As of the writing of this book, there are no published studies showing that you can get too much omega-3, although there's no need to overdo it.

Incidentally, if you are a strict vegetarian or if you are allergic to fish, you can also get omega-3 from such plant sources as walnuts, flax, chia seeds, canola oil, and even algae. There are several suppliers. Just search "vegetarian omega-3" on the Internet and you'll find plenty of sources. There is a catch, however: Plant sources of omega-3s are "short chain," abbreviated ALA, for alpha linolenic acid. These are good, but not great sources of omega-3. Humans don't do a very good job converting ALA into EPA and DHA (roughly 5% conversion rate), so although ALA is technically an omega-3 fat, it's not nearly as beneficial as EPA and DHA. When buying a food product that makes the claim "Now with omega-3," be sure to read the label. More times than not, it will contain a very low level of ALA, so you're probably not getting the bang you are expecting. (My rule of thumb is that if any manufactured product offers a health claim on the label, it's usually trying to hide something!)

One thing to keep in mind regarding omega-3: Not all fish and not all fish oils are created equal. Table 1 shows a list of the EPA and DHA levels of most types of fish. (Table 1 is courtesy of Bill Harris, PhD, one of the world's leading authorities on omega-3s and the codeveloper of the HS-Omega-3 Index.)

By increasing your intake of omega-3 (specifically EPA+DHA), either through fatty fish or fish oil supplements, you will increase your HS-Omega-3 Index. There are many reasons why it makes sense to have a healthy omega-3 level. Reducing your risk of death from coronary heart disease is just a start.

Between fish and omega-3 supplements, I consume about 3,000–4,000 mg of EPA+DHA per day. At last check, my HS Omega-3 Index was 9.1%, which puts me in the "desirable" range. I tell people all the time that when it comes to omega-3, I want to be Japanese! Table 2 explains why.

Thanks to Dr. Bill Harris and his research partner, Dr. Clemens von Schacky, it's now fairly easy to get your HS-Omega-3 Index measured. Check with your doctor to see if he or she has a relationship with HDL Labs out of Richmond, Virginia. If so, your test will often be covered by insurance. If not, you can have your HS-Omega-3 Index measured with a finger-stick test-kit. For more information, visit www.omegaquant.com.

Table 1. EPA and DHA Levels by Fish Type

Fish and Seafood	EPA	DHA	EPA+DHA
	per 3oz (85 g) serving		
Chum Salmon (canned)	402	597	999
Rainbow Trout (farmed)	284	697	981
Coho Salmon (wild)	341	559	900
Sardines (canned)	402	433	835
Albacore (or White) Tuna (canned)	198	535	733
Shark (raw)	267	444	711
Swordfish	117	579	696
Sea Bass	175	473	648
Halibut	77	318	395
Oysters (farmed)	195	179	374
King Crab	251	100	351
Walleye	93	245	338
Dungeness Crab	239	96	335
Scallops	141	169	310
Skipjack Tuna	77	201	278
Mixed Shrimp	145	122	267
Clams	117	124	241
Yellowfin Tuna	40	197	237
Light Chunk Tuna (canned)	40	190	230
Catfish (wild)	85	116	201
Catfish (farmed)	42	109	151
Cod	3	131	134
Mahi-Mahi (dolphin fish)	22	96	118
Tilapia	4	111	115
Orange Roughy	5	21	26

Source: Bill Harris, PhD

Table 2. Percentage of EPA+DHA in Red Blood Cells

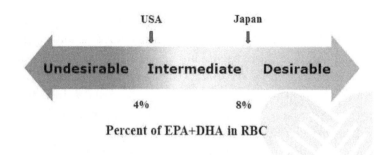

Source: Bill Harris, PhD.

Vitamin D

The next item on my nutritional supplement list is vitamin D. This nutrient is so important that I consider it right under omega-3, like number 1A rather than number 2. Did you know that vitamin D is not even a vitamin? When it was first identified in the early 1900s, it behaved much like a vitamin, hence the name, but it's actually a steroid hormone. The human body makes vitamin D when the UVB light from the sun hits our skin. This is why vitamin D is often referred to as the sunshine vitamin. Exposure to sun triggers a process whereby the body manufactures, or synthesizes, vitamin D in the kidneys and liver.

We learned about vitamin D because of its relationship with rickets, a condition in which children's bones don't properly calcify. This was a very common problem during the Industrial Revolution, when many kids weren't getting much sun exposure. It's estimated that in 1900, 80 percent of the children in Boston had rickets. As soon as they spent some time in the sun or got a minimal dose of vitamin D from cod liver oil, however, the condition almost immediately went away. In the 1930s, most dairies started fortifying milk with vitamin D, and the rickets epidemic was eradicated. Believe it or not, for a while, you could even find vitamin D in beer!

It turns out that vitamin D is related to much more than bone health. It actually plays a developmental role in about 10 percent of the human genome. According to the July 2007 issue of the *New England Journal of Medicine*, thousands of research articles link vitamin D deficiency to a wide variety of issues, including arthritis, cardiovascular disease, depression, chronic pain, age-related macular degeneration, cancers (including breast, ovarian, prostate, pancreatic, stomach, and more), osteoporosis, hypertension, Alzheimer's disease, diabetes, and immunity. A 2009 study in the *Archives of Internal Medicine* showed that those with the lowest levels of vitamin D are 36 percent more likely to suffer from colds, flu, and upper respiratory tract infections.

The problem is this: 77 percent of American adolescents and adults are deficient or insufficient in vitamin D, meaning the level of vitamin D in their blood is below 30 ng/ml. It also appears that our vitamin D levels are dropping. According to data from the Centers for Disease Control's National Health and Nutrition Examination Survey, between 1988 and 2004, Americans' average blood levels of vitamin D dropped 6 ng/ml. There are several explanations for this. One is that most Americans live inside and work inside, so we don't get consistent exposure to the sun. Another is that Americans are getting bigger. Vitamin D is fat soluble, so when an individual's BMI goes up, vitamin D gets diluted in the additional adipose tissue. Another suspected reason for the drop in average vitamin D levels is the use of sunscreen. An SPF (sun protection factor) of 15 or greater blocks 99 percent of the synthesis of vitamin D, according to the July 19, 2007, issue of the *New England Journal of Medicine*. The same UVB light that triggers the production of vitamin D also causes sunburn. Although I certainly don't advocate going without sunscreen, I caution you not to throw the baby out with the bathwater. Dr. Edward Giovannucci of Harvard, in a 2006 issue of the *Journal of the National*

Cancer Institute, has suggested that "sunlight might prevent thirty deaths for each one caused by skin cancer."

The only way for you to know your vitamin D level is to get it checked with a blood test. Although many doctors now routinely check vitamin D levels, you may need to ask for this test. Be specific and ask for a 25(OH)D test (pronounced 25 hydroxy D), as opposed to a test called 1,25(OH)2D. I've seen the price of a vitamin D test vary from less than $100 to more than $350. Sometimes the test is covered by insurance, and sometimes it's not. There are also in-home test kits available from a number of organizations, including the Vitamin D Council ($58, www.vitamindcouncil.org) and ZRT Labs in Beaverton, Oregon ($75, www.zrtlab.com).

The generally accepted "sufficient" range for vitamin D is a blood level of 30–100 ng/ml (vitamin D is also sometimes expressed as nmol/L; 1 ng/ml = 2.5 nmol/L, and 1 nmol/L = 0.4 ng/ml). A level of 21–29 is considered insufficient, and a level less than 20 is considered deficient. Vitamin D toxicity is defined as a blood level greater than 150 ng/ml and is extremely uncommon. Most Americans (including adults, adolescents, and children) have blood levels below 30 ng/ml, so if you get tested, do not be surprised to find that your blood level is low. If it's very low, often, a doctor will put you on a prescription vitamin D. Most of the time, this will be 50,000 IU to be taken once, twice, or sometimes three times a week. This is referred to as a hyperdose intended to quickly boost your vitamin D level into an appropriate range.

The question of what constitutes the ideal blood level for vitamin D is hotly debated. I encourage you to talk to your doctor about this, although most people are told that anything above 30 is fine. I'm not a physician, but I have attended multiple vitamin D conferences, interviewed many of the leading researchers, and read a great deal of the published studies. My personal opinion is that I want my blood level to hover somewhere in the 40–60 ng/ml range. This is what I strive for, but you should discuss your particular needs with your doctor. If you get your vitamin D tested and it's where you would like it to be, just keep doing what you're doing. If your level is low, but not low enough to require a prescription, you generally have two options: more sun exposure or vitamin D supplements, as it's extremely hard to get enough vitamin D from food alone.

Vitamin D in supplement form is available as vitamin D2 or D3. Most of the research indicates that D3 is the most bioavailable, although one study by vitamin D guru Dr. Michael Holick suggests that they are equally efficacious. I generally don't hang my hat on just one study, but because Dr. Holick is so well regarded in this space, I'll take his word for it. Most of the vitamin D supplements you find at the pharmacy, grocery store, or health food store will be vitamin D3.

Unlike omega-3 products, vitamin D is a commodity. I suggest you buy the cheapest you can find. Just make sure you take enough. There is a six-fold variability in how different people respond to D, but when you assess all of the research, it seems as if 2,000 IU of vitamin D daily is a pretty good place to start. Again, we are all different, so make sure you speak with your healthcare provider. There are many factors that influence our vitamin D status, including sun exposure, time of year (in North America, there is more UVB light available in the summer than in the winter), BMI, age, latitude, and complexion.

Considering a Multivitamin

The question of whether it makes sense to take a daily multivitamin is an interesting one. Some studies show benefit, while others do not. There are several things to consider. First, not all multivitamins are created equal. There is enormous variability in both the nutrients included in each particular formula and, more important, in the *amount* (dose) of the particular nutrients. This can be extremely confusing for someone who doesn't pay a great deal of attention to the topic. I often joke with audiences that the average American doesn't know the difference between a milligram, a microgram, or a telegram . . . not to mention an international unit! The proper range—what's sometimes referred to as the therapeutic window—is critical.

A perfect example of this is with the nutrient lutein, which is a carotenoid found in kale, spinach, turnip greens, and collards. Lutein is a wonderful nutrient for the eyes, especially the macula, in the center of the retina. Multiple studies have shown that having healthy levels of lutein in the eyes can lower risk of age-related macular degeneration, dry eyes, and cataracts, and can even help with the visual performance of athletes by improving glare recovery and temporal processing speeds (for more on this, see Chapter 27, "Batter Up! Vision Is Where It All Starts"). The challenge, though, is in knowing how much lutein you need. Most of the studies indicate that the optimum daily dose is at least 6 milligrams (mg); however, when you read the label of many multivitamins, if they include lutein at all, it's often only 250 micrograms (mcg)—only 1/24 what the research shows is most beneficial.

The reason for this is simple: economics. Lutein is a pretty expensive ingredient, and if manufacturers add more to the product, they either need to raise their price or lower their profit margin. Neither of these options makes good business sense. Is including a "pixie dust" amount of an ingredient in a product legal? Sure! Is it ethical? You be the judge of that.

Multivitamins are not created equal, and neither are the studies about multivitamins. Negative studies routinely are the only ones that get reported in the mainstream (i.e., nonscientific) press, which makes sense, because to get our attention, media outlets need to shock or scare us. Small, short studies of unhealthy people taking a multivitamin should not be expected to show reduction of cancer, heart attacks, dementia, and so on. There is a tremendous difference between a short observational study versus a large, double-blind, placebo-controlled clinical trial, however. The latter is hard to find in the world of supplements because it's not required by law and because quality research is both time-consuming and expensive.

There are obviously hundreds of supplement companies to choose from, and some are better than others. I encourage you to find a manufacturer with a proven track record and, ideally, with a commitment to research. I don't believe that a product that offers only RDA (recommended daily allowance) levels of ingredients provides much benefit. The RDA levels help prevent such vitamin-deficiency diseases as scurvy, pellagra, and beriberi but generally aren't enough to have much impact on diabetes, heart disease or stroke. Also, be aware that the "expert" at the health food or vitamin store may or may not be incented to direct you toward a particular brand. They often are "spiffed" (compensated) when they can get you to buy one product over another. I prefer to buy supplements online to get the best value.

Supplements: The Bottom Line

In addition to omega-3 and vitamin D, I think of multivitamins as an insurance policy: It helps me cover my bases. I make every effort possible to get the majority of my nutrition from my diet, but my supplements help "just in case." Ideally, your diet should include a wide variety of fruits and green, leafy vegetables, healthy protein and fat, whole grains, and plenty of nuts, seeds, and fresh berries. I view proper supplementation as just an added bonus!

"Eat fish, not hot dogs."
– Dr. Joseph Hibbeln

"If it came from a plant, eat it.
If it was made in a plant, don't."
– Michael Pollan

27.

Batter Up! Vision Is Where It All Starts

Imagine this: It's late afternoon on a beautiful summer day. You're in the batter's box, facing 6'5" major league pitcher Yu Darvish. The setting sun is casting a distinct shadow that falls halfway between the pitcher's mound and home plate. Running through your mind is "What type of pitch will Darvish throw?" Will it be a 97-mph fastball or a 63-mph curve?

It takes no more than half a second for a pitch thrown at 80 mph to reach the plate, so you won't have much time to make your decision. In just a fraction of a second, your eyes must evaluate the speed, direction, and anticipated path of the pitch. That visual data is passed through the optic nerve and into the brain, which sends a signal through your nerves to your muscles to immediately react to the information being processed. This all hinges on your hand-eye coordination, which can mean the difference between a game-winning base hit or game-ending strikeout. This entire process is obviously highly dependent on vision.

What if there were a way to improve your processing speed by 15 percent? As an athlete, would that increase your odds of success? What if you could also improve your ability to handle glare (by 58 percent), enhance your contrast sensitivity (as in picking up the flight of a baseball against a blue sky or green backdrop), and increase your visual range by approximately 30 percent? In nearly every sport, the ability to see better and react more quickly results in improved performance. Consider in football the expectation for a quarterback to instantly determine whether to throw to one of three different receivers, dump a pass off to a running back, or tuck and run. Or for a receiver or defensive back, while running at full speed, to leap in traffic, then locate the pass in bright sunshine or against glaring stadium lights, and then react to a tipped ball to make the catch. A spike in volleyball can top 90 mph, a slap shot in hockey often exceeds 100 mph, and serves in tennis routinely reach 124 mph for women and 140 mph for men (Andy Roddick's serve was once recorded at 155 mph!).

Nutrition's Role in Enhancing Visual Performance

As it turns out, nutrition plays an incredible role in how an athlete's eyes perform during competition. Research from the 1990s shows that lutein and zeaxanthin, carotenoids found at high levels in kale and spinach, can help lower the risk of age-related macular degeneration, the leading cause of blindness in adults over sixty-five. Current research shows that these two nutrients, when delivered in the proper doses, can also improve the visual performance of athletes. A 2008 trial published in *Optometry and Vision Science* studied forty healthy men and women with a mean age of 23.9 years. After four months of supplementation with 10 mg of lutein and 2 mg of zeaxanthin, their glare recovery improved significantly. After six months, the subjects' ability to tolerate glaring light had improved 58 percent, and the time to recover their sight following exposure to bright light (known as photostress) improved by five seconds, or 14 percent.

We all have experienced how our eyes need time to adjust when going from a brightly lit lobby into a dark movie theater, or what happens while driving at night when an oncoming car or truck passes us with the bright headlights on.

Internal Sunglasses

The back part of the eye is the retina; in the center of the retina is the macula. All vision hinges on the ability for light, whether it be natural or artificial, to pass into the brain via the optic nerve once it has entered the eye. The light needs to be filtered, which is a primary role of the macula. In fact, the macula has been described as the eye's internal sunglasses. As it turns out, there is a very high concentration of lutein and its sister molecule zeaxanthin in the macula. That concentration, or density, can be objectively measured by something called macular pigment (MP). MP is a function of your diet; the more foods you eat that contain lutein (e.g., kale, spinach, turnip greens, and collards), the higher your MP will be.

According to Dr. Paul Bernstein from the Moran Eye Center at the University of Utah, a leading researcher of macular degeneration, the average American consumes about 1–1.5 mg of lutein per day. That's not much. Most of us are not consuming enough servings of lutein-containing foods. (When was the last time you had a big serving of kale?) Upping your intake of lutein, whether from food or supplements, will increase your MP, which will in turn improve your visual performance. The dose that the research shows provides a measurable benefit is 10 mg of lutein plus 2 mg of zeaxanthin.

A 2012 study published in the *American Journal of Clinical Nutrition* showed that lutein and zeaxanthin "shorten photostress recovery times, enhance chromatic contrast, and increase visual range. In addition, it appears that these important nutrients might also increase temporal processing speeds." For example, an athlete with a higher MP concentration would have faster temporal vision, allowing for more "snapshots" to be taken in a fixed amount of time. The study's authors noted that "faster temporal processing speed would facilitate faster reaction times, thus enabling quicker decisions (e.g., whether or not to swing at the pitch)."

Pelé's Exceptional Exteroception

On a 2013 trip to Brazil, I met with Professor Oscar Erichsen, the head trainer of Atletico Paranaense, one of the country's premier soccer teams. He recalled in great detail something that happened in the 1970 World Cup played in Mexico City: During one of the Brazilian matches, Pelé, arguably the best soccer player in history, took a shot on goal from midfield. The shot sailed wide, but the mere fact that Pelé had even attempted such a feat sent shockwaves throughout the soccer world. That had never happened before on such a large stage. Professor Oscar explained that the shot attempt was significant for two reasons. One was the obvious leg strength that it took to launch such a blast. The other was more subtle.

Pelé had an incredible ability to constantly evaluate data in the throes of competition: How were his teammates positioned in comparison to the opponents? How fast was defender A compared to defender B? How did the length of the grass and the direction of the wind affect the flight of the ball? On this particular play, Pelé sensed that the defenders nearest him were out of position and that the opposing goalie had drifted away from the net. In an instant, he made the decision to take a shot that, despite being off-line, fans still talk about more than forty-five years later.

Scientifically, the ability to read one's external environment is known as exteroception. Professor Oscar said no one has ever had better exteroception than Pelé. We often hear about excellent exteroception in descriptions of skilled point guards in basketball ("He has eyes in the back of his head") or in successful quarterbacks on the gridiron ("The game just seems to slow down for them").

Superior hand-eye (or in the case of soccer players, foot-eye) coordination must start with superior vision. Sport-specific drills can improve coordination, muscle memory, and reaction times, but proper nutrition also plays a significant role in performance. Lutein and zeaxanthin (6-10 mg/day), along with such nutrients as omega-3 fats (at least 1,000 mg of EPA+DHA/day) and vitamin D (at least 2,000 IU /day) in the appropriate doses can help maximize potential. (For additional information on these important supplements, see chapter 26, "What About Supplements?"). The infamous military leader, Napoleon Bonaparte, believed that "an army marches on its stomach." He knew that just the slightest improvement can often mean the difference between victory and defeat.

> "Success is piece of mind which is a direct result of knowing you did you best to become the best you are capable of becoming."
> – John Wooden

"People often say that motivation doesn't last.
Well, neither does bathing –
that's why we recommend it daily."

– Zig Ziglar

28.

Motivation: Catch It While You Can!

As we discussed in Chapter 21, Stanford researcher B. J. Fogg believes three things need to be present at the same time for any behavior to take place: a trigger (call to action), ability (skill), and motivation. Of these three, Dr. Fogg says, motivation is the *least* important. That may come as a surprise to you, given how much attention is paid to motivation by our society.

When we are truly motivated, we are capable of all sorts of things, but there is a big difference between compliance and long-term behavior (i.e., habits). Compliance is the act of conforming, acquiescing, or yielding. It's something we usually do in the short term. It's relatively easy to do something once or twice or for a limited amount of time. Most weight-loss diets are a perfect example of compliance: You decide you are going to dramatically alter your usual pattern of eating with the goal of losing a fixed amount of weight. It may be incredibly challenging, even painful, but if you're motivated, you're often able to accomplish what you set out to do, because you know it won't last forever.

Motivation, however, is often in a state of flux. Adopting new behaviors is much easier when motivation is high. But then life happens and motivation tends to wane. It would be great to figure out how to stay motivated all the time, but that's impossible. Motivation is elusive. I love what social ecologist Peter Drucker said about it: "We know nothing about motivation. All we can do is write books about it."

So, if weight loss is your initial goal and source of motivation, what will sustain the weight loss once you've hit your target (the maintenance phase)? Healthy habits. As you know, habits are something you don't have to think about. Habits happen whether your motivation is high or low (like brushing your teeth or putting on your seat belt). To build healthy habits, we need to have a specific plan, leverage triggers, and build skills. Be patient. Change is a process. My suggestion is to take advantage of motivation but not to depend on it.

Surrounding yourself with motivated people can be very helpful. This is why group exercise classes or activities can be so beneficial for some people. In his book *The Power of Habit*, Charles Duhigg writes, "For a habit to stay changed, people must believe change is possible and most often that belief only emerges with the help of a group." Humans are social beings so it helps to interact with like-minded people who have like-minded goals. Weight loss is one thing, but if your objective is to permanently embrace a healthy lifestyle that will result in feeling better, looking better, and dramatically lowering your risk of disease and disability, concentrate on building healthy habits. Look at motivation as fuel for your fire. What motivates you?

"Impossible is not a fact, it's an opinion."

"The entire population of the universe, with one trifling exception, is composed of others."

– John Andrew Holmes

29.

Broadening the Scope from "What about Me?" to "What about Us?"

I spoke one morning to a large group of human resource (HR) professionals at a conference in southern Texas. The topic was "How to Take Your Wellness Program to the Next Level." Ostensibly, the talk detailed how to introduce next-generation wellness opportunities in corporate environments. I also included suggestions about how the attendees could improve their own personal health. I pointed out that despite sharing the planet with nearly eight billion people, no one has more impact on one's own health than oneself. Each of us has the ability to affect our own future more than any doctor, employer, spouse, friend, or government program ever could. No one else can eat for us, exercise for us, sleep for us, or manage stress for us. We have to do it for ourselves. In other words, as I often say, your health cannot be outsourced.

After my talk, there was a fifteen-minute break before the next presenter. Several people came to the stage to ask questions before I packed up my stuff and headed out of the conference room. As I made my way to the door, I was approached by a woman I would guess to be in her early thirties. She was short, well-dressed, and a bit overweight. She had tears in her eyes. She thanked me for the talk and for providing her with a wakeup call. During the talk, she said, she came to a major realization: She was very much at risk for serious health problems. My message had motivated her to finally take charge of her health. I gave her a hug and encouraged her not to be so hard on herself.

It's important to remember that our future is much more important than our past. Don't trip over things behind you.

As we spoke, I learned that this woman was the HR director for about 120 employees for a small city in Central Texas. I asked if the city had a structured wellness program. She said it did not, but what really got my attention was the reason why. She had not implemented any corporate wellness initiatives because she was embarrassed about her own size. She felt that the other employees would view her as a hypocrite for promoting a program that she herself was not embracing. As gently as possible, I looked her in the eye and told her that, although her feelings were understandable, she was being very selfish. As the HR director, she was in a unique position to positively influence a large group of people; she alone had the opportunity to not just improve lives but actually *save* lives. The woman was obviously taken aback by such a direct assessment. Unfortunately, I sensed it wasn't going to change her attitude at all.

As humans, we are wired to ask ourselves the same question hundreds of times per day: *How is this going to affect me?* We usually don't consciously verbalize the question, but when we hear or learn something new from a friend or colleague, or when we read about something in the newspaper or online, we naturally wonder how we as individuals will be affected. This is not a commentary on the selfish nature of humans; it's just my takeaway from decades of observation—including plenty of self-observation. For example, living in North Texas, the weather can often be life-threatening. Destructive storms move across the state in large vertical bands that usually track from west to east. If I flip on the radio or TV and learn that severe weather is headed my way in the Dallas/Fort Worth area, I pay *much* more attention than if the weather is going to bypass the area. A tsunami in Singapore or an earthquake in Japan has a much different effect on me than does a threatening tornado in North Texas. Here's another example: I drive a Toyota. If I learn that Ford or Chevrolet has just recalled 20,000 cars because of some sort of defect, I tune out because that simply doesn't affect me, but if Toyota were to announce a recall, I'd be all ears! It's simply the way we're wired.

But here's a radical idea: I encourage you to consider thinking a bit more broadly. Although you might not be all that interested in going for a walk or in making a healthy choice when eating out, think about how your behavior might be influencing those around you. Although most humans tend to be somewhat self-centered (evolutionarily speaking, our survival depended on this trait!), I believe that we are all on Earth to have a positive effect on other people. You have a much greater influence on those around you than you might think. (Remember the study in Chapter 21 – that showed the BMI of your friends has a much greater effect than that of your spouse on your own BMI.)

This concept is even more important for those who are in a position of leadership—parents, teachers, coaches, supervisors, managers, and especially CEOs. We have the ability to influence those around us, and this influence can be either positive or negative. Take the time to evaluate your role in other people's lives—it's an enlightening exercise. Leading by example is powerful. As a parent, I'm convinced that kids pay far more attention to what we *do* than what we *say*. Whether it's in your home, school, church, or the HR department of a small Texas town, find a way to model and promote healthy behavior. And remember that you don't have to be a pillar of health to get started. Baby steps taken in the right direction can really add up! Instead of asking, "What about me?" let's consider "What about us?"

"It always seems impossible until it's done."
– Nelson Mandela

"The power of one, if fearless and focused, is formidable,
but the power of many working together is better."
– Gloria Macapagal Arroyo

30.

Corporate Wellness: Obligation or Opportunity?

Author's note: Heads up! This chapter is intended for leaders interested in ways to influence employee health in a work environment.

An effective CEO shouldn't spend too much time worrying about today—or even tomorrow, for that matter. CEOs need to gaze out the window and ask, "How should I be preparing my organization for the next five to ten years?" Obviously, managing employee healthcare should be a primary concern, but what about employee *health*?

The term "wellness program" has come a long way in the past decade. It wasn't long ago that whenever the term was mentioned, most people responded with furrowed brows and asked, "What's that?" Today, it's a different story. Now, when a wellness program is referenced, more times than not, the response is a nod followed by "Oh yeah, we have one of those!"

For many companies, wellness programs are now par for the course, much like water coolers, holiday parties, and 401(k)s. The problem is that not all wellness programs are created equal. In fact, studies show that many of them don't make much of a difference. That's right, the majority of wellness programs are a waste of time and resources! Most, but certainly not all. So, what makes for a successful wellness program? I believe there are five mandatory requirements, and the first one may be a bit surprising.

1. Stop Calling It a Wellness Program!

To be honest, companies encourage employees to be healthier to boost workforce productivity and save money. The driving force is economics, not philanthropy. There's nothing wrong with that transparency. Unfortunately, generating a profit has become more difficult in light of double-digit increases in healthcare costs each year.

What does "wellness" even mean? "Wellness program" is a vague term that is not applied in an impactful manner in most employer benefits programs. The typical wellness program includes lunch-and-learns, fruit and vegetable challenges, in-office massage days and fun runs. These activities are fine, and can certainly contribute to the overall culture and morale of an organization, but if the goal is to improve the troops' health, it's imperative that the program be laser-focused on *measurable outcomes.* That means prioritizing and incentivizing initiatives that will make a difference and then measuring the results!

Instead of "wellness program," HR leaders and corporate decision makers should consider the more useful and descriptive term "clinical improvement program." Why? Because it all boils down to reversing risk factors—especially those that lead to such diseases as diabetes, obesity (yes, the American Medical Association has defined obesity as a disease), arthritis, depression, heart disease, and cancer. If the "wellness" efforts are not measurably improving clinical risk factors of the workforce, then the organization is simply spinning its wheels.

2. Look in the Mirror

What kind of company are you leading? One that's willing to create a culture that holds employees *accountable* for their behavior? Or one that's interested in offering options that may not be embraced by the workforce? If it's the latter, understand that this type of culture won't do much to slow the production and progression of disease. This kind of culture also won't generate much, if any, impact on clinical risk factors, improving employee health or reducing healthcare costs.

If a company really wants to move the needle on workforce health, it's imperative that leadership engages in honest dialog. Be willing to ask some tough questions to determine the organization's core beliefs concerning its role in healthcare. For example, which of the statements below best reflect the organization's beliefs?

As an employer, the limit of the company's role is to provide access to market-competitive health insurance and to share in paying the cost.
OR
As a provider of health benefits, it is the company's responsibility to influence personal behavior and medical outcomes.

There is no right or wrong answer, and it's likely your organization exists somewhere in between these two extremes. The goal of examining your organization's healthcare beliefs is to help leadership define rights and roles. Here's another comparison of statements to help an organization define its healthcare position:

It is part of HR's job to design and administer benefits, but health status is a private matter.
OR
It is part of HR's job to improve the health of employees and covered dependents.

Remember, the only way to improve corporate health is to get individuals to change the behaviors that affect the risk factors we know lead to health insurance claims. If an individual has skin in the game, the odds improve dramatically for that person to make a positive change. It ultimately boils down to accountability. Think about an individual's driving habits. If someone knows that getting a speeding ticket won't cost them a dime, that person will most likely not think twice about driving too fast. The same concept applies to personal health: If someone else is paying for the office visit, acid reflux medication, or bypass surgery, an individual is going to be much less likely to skip donuts for breakfast or go for a walk.

For some companies, individual accountability is an easy concept to embrace and leadership understands that the status quo is not a sustainable option. They recognize that employees must be part of their own healthcare decisions. Other companies fear the fallout, however; they believe their employees will complain and that morale will suffer. But effective employee buy-in is often just a matter of how the message is communicated. Most employees today understand that their behavior influences their health and that they have to be more personally accountable, so messaging and strategy are critical.

3. Assess the Problem

If an organization has 100 employees and the workforce reflects national averages for health states, then at least seventy-five employees would be considered overweight, forty out of that total would be categorized as obese (a body mass index above thirty), twelve would have diabetes (three of whom don't know it yet), and thirty-seven would qualify as prediabetic (this is an important number, as the clock is ticking steadily closer to diabetes!). About half of the population would have high blood pressure, seventeen would have high cholesterol, thirty-three would have high triglycerides, fifteen would smoke, about seventy-five would fail to get enough physical activity, sixty-two would have sleep issues, seventy-seven would struggle with stress, nine would suffer from depression, and forty-one would live with chronic pain. All companies and their employees are unique, but most reflect these national averages.

To be sure, it's extremely helpful to collect aggregate workforce data, which requires biometric screenings of employees annually. These screenings need to include height, weight, waist circumference, a simple survey of family history (i.e., incidences of cancer, heart disease, stroke, diabetes, etc.), depression, tobacco use, and blood pressure. Screenings should include a fasting blood analysis that measures cholesterol (including HDL and LDL), triglycerides, blood glucose, and (for those who qualify) hemoglobin A1c, which looks at average blood sugar over the past two or three months. The biometric screening can be done either in a doctor's office or during an onsite assessment.

Screenings are often done during open enrollment or at an annual corporate health fair. Participation in annual screenings might allow employees to receive a discount on their health insurance premiums (up to 50 percent, which is a very powerful incentive). One of the most important lessons from a biometric screening is, in the aggregate, how many employees have diabetes or prediabetes. The outcomes can be shocking. The cost of healthcare for someone with diabetes is at least *twice* that of someone without the disease. The real opportunity to influence both the health of the employees and the cost of healthcare is to keep those with prediabetes from "converting" to diabetes. More than 90 percent of people with diabetes have type 2 diabetes, which is primarily a lifestyle disease attributed to both obesity and physical inactivity. In other words, it's preventable! From the perspective of a clinical-improvement initiative (aka wellness program), this is the low-hanging fruit.

An excellent predictor of diabetic risk is metabolic syndrome (MetS), a cluster of conditions including increased blood pressure, high blood glucose, excessive body fat around the waist, elevated HDL cholesterol, and elevated triglycerides. Together, these conditions dramatically increase the risk of heart disease, stroke, and diabetes (by as much as 2,100 percent). When an individual has three or more of these factors out of range, by definition, that person has MetS. It's estimated that at least 25 percent of adults in the

United States have MetS, and it's closer to 50 percent for those over the age of fifty. This reality exemplifies why it's critical for a company to accurately assess the health of its workforce. Unless risk is objectively measured, it's impossible to know how many serious, and expensive, illnesses lie in wait.

4. Have a Definitive Strategy

Once risk is determined through initial health assessments, it's possible for the company to develop a strategic game plan. By combining aggregate biometric workforce data with demographics and claims history, companies can accurately predict their future healthcare costs. Leadership can then design a plan that will not only improve employee health, but also flatten the cost curve.

The cost of healthcare ultimately boils down to two factors: utilization and price. To effectively move the needle on healthcare costs, both factors must be addressed. Aggressively working to improve the health of the workforce will result in lower utilization of healthcare (that is, employees simply won't need to have as many "-ectomies"). Lower utilization will happen only if the organization positively affects the appropriate risk factors. For instance, if only 3 percent of the workforce smokes, then investing in a smoking-cessation program is not a good use of resources. If a significant percentage of the workforce has MetS, then a MetS risk reversal program is an excellent place to start. Multiple solutions are available for employers to measurably improve the health of their workforces, so be sure to look for wellness programs that are scalable, easy to implement, and offer clinical results. Don't hesitate to ask for performance guarantees.

It's also critical to focus on what an organization is paying for medical procedures and services. There are several stakeholders in the healthcare equation: patients (employees), employers, doctors, hospitals, insurers, and the government. Obviously, not all of these stakeholders are aligned. For a variety of reasons, the amount that patients ultimately end up paying has always been somewhat of a mystery. Although the idea of asking the doctor, insurance company, or hospital what a procedure will cost before having it done has been almost unheard of in the past, that's changing in a hurry. Because both employees and employers now often have skin in the game, it makes sense for both stakeholder groups to cost-compare before booking an appointment. For example, in North Texas, the cost of a simple MRI can vary from $640 to $1,900, depending on where the service is delivered. The variance for a CT scan is $540 to $2,600. In-network knee replacement in North Texas (one of the most expensive regions of the country for healthcare) can vary from $29,400 to $57,500, depending on the facility. Obviously, cost comparisons offer a tremendous opportunity for savings for both the health consumer/customer and their company.

Additionally, there is very little correlation between quality and price. Many times, the lowest-priced option for a particular service or procedure also has the best customer-satisfaction scores, along with the lowest complication and re-admission rates. Until recently, this type of information was not available to the patient/customer, but now, price transparency is saving some companies millions of dollars. Taking advantage of proven solutions is easy, and the benefits are immediate.

5. Rely on Experts

The key to any successful clinical-improvement program is dovetailing it with the organization's health plan. Companies often have benefits programs that include healthcare coverage and then a separate wellness program. That's a mistake; the two must be integrated. Although compliant wellness programs have been sanctioned by law since the 1990s, there have recently been some advantageous changes for employers. As of January 1, 2014, employers can charge a 30 percent differential on healthcare premiums based on such outcomes as body mass index, cholesterol, blood pressure, blood glucose, and other biometrics. The law allows for a 50 percent differential for smokers. This gives employers a tremendous ability to hold employees accountable, but employers must follow the rules established by HIPAA (Health Insurance Portability and Accountability Act), GINA (Genetic Information Nondiscrimination Act), the ADA (Americans with Disabilities Act), ERISA (Employee Retirement Income Security Act), and so on. HIPAA privacy issues matter for companies of all sizes, but can be a particular challenge for smaller organizations.

Healthcare costs have been rising for years, and the worst is most likely yet to come. For company leadership, there are really only two choices: stand by and pretend that everything is going to be fine, or evaluate the options and develop clinical-improvement plans that will *measurably* improve the physical health of the workforce and the fiscal health of the organization.

> "A human being is happiest and most successful when dedicated to a cause outside his own individual selfish satisfaction."
> – Dr. Benjamin Spock

"Do or do not. There is no try."
- Yoda

31.

Here Comes the Tsunami!

There are three kinds of lies: lies, damned lies, and statistics. The great American humorist Mark Twain often gets credit for that statement, although it most likely originated in England in the late 1800s. Whatever the origin, the takeaway is simple: Statistics can be manipulated to support or detract from just about any position or argument. One position that has not been subject to manipulation is the increasing number of Americans living with diabetes. February is American Heart Month, a federally-designated event to remind Americans to focus on heart health. Each year, right around Valentine's Day, we are inundated with dire statistics regarding heart disease. It kills more Americans than any other disease; 750,000 Americans will have a heart attack this year; and 70 percent of heart disease is preventable. Although these numbers are all true, they are old news. Deaths from heart disease have actually decreased dramatically over the past fifty years in the United States. What we really need to be paying attention to is how rapidly the rate of diabetes is exploding!

When someone passes away, the official death certificate has to include the cause of death. The problem is, it's rare that someone dies from a single health issue. What if an individual is obese; is physically inactive; smokes; and has heart disease, diabetes, hypertension, or cancer; and they suffer a fatal stroke? What should the attending physician list as the cause of death? That's an important question, because multiple factors (comorbidities) were obviously at play.

From 1997 to 2011, for adults ages thirty to eighty-four, only 3.3 percent of death certificates listed diabetes as the underlying cause of death. A study published in the January 25, 2017, edition of *PLOS ONE* indicates that number should be closer to 12 percent, which would move diabetes from the seventh-leading cause of death to the third (behind heart disease and cancer).

At first glance, those numbers might not cause any alarm, but let's look downfield. As previously mentioned, more than 90 percent of diabetes cases are classified as type 2, which is primarily a function of obesity and physical inactivity. In other words, it's preventable. The prevalence of diabetes in the United States has *tripled* between 1976 and 2017. More alarming, it's predicted that at least 40 percent of Americans born after the year 2000 will develop diabetes (up from the current 12.3 percent of adults ages twenty and older). Yes, you read that right: 40 percent! If that does not have your attention, consider the economic cost! The *Journal of the American Medical Association* published a study in December 2016 of the ten most costly health expenses (see figure below). The cost of diabetes is at the top of the list, at more than $101 billion a year! Even more startling, the cost of health expenses related to diabetes is growing *thirty-six times faster* than the number-two condition, which is ischemic heart disease.

10 Most Costly Hearth Expenses

(2013)

• Diabetes (36x)	$101.4 b
• Ischemic heart disease	$88.1
• Low back and neck pain	$87.6
• Hypertension	$83.9
• Injuries from falls	$76.3
• Depressive disorders	$71.1
• Oral related problems	$66.4
• Vision and hearing problems	$59.0
• Skin-related problems	$55.7
• Pregnancy and postpartum care	$55.6

Institute of Health Metrics and Evaluation (U.W.), December 27, 2016 (JAMA)

What does all this mean? Well, as my dad used to say, we're in deep yogurt! From a health perspective, where we've *been* is interesting and where we *are* is important, but where we're *going* is frightening. Although we can outsource many things in our lives—laundry, meal preparation, lawn care, and so on—we simply cannot outsource our health. Individually and collectively, Americans must recognize that most cases of diabetes could be avoided. If we don't correct course soon, no one is going to have a checkbook big enough to pay for what's coming.

"One person can make a difference. Be that person."
- Wyland

"If you ask me what I came into this life to do,
I will tell you: I came to live out loud."
– Emile Zola

32.

Squaring off the Curve: Exceptional Survival

If you've ever heard Dr. Ken Cooper speak, you've probably heard the expression "squaring off the curve." What he means is that we should strive to live a long and healthy life to the fullest and then . . . die suddenly! When people hear that explained for the first time, they often laugh nervously. Should this be the goal? Of course! What's the alternative? Slowly fading into the sunset in an old-folks home with a stranger wiping applesauce off of your chin?

As it turns out, "just hanging on" is the way most Americans spend the final years of their lives; they are *alive* but not really *living*. The data show that somewhere between 93 percent and 97 percent of us live what could be described as high-risk lifestyles; as a result, our final years are often spent just surviving, possibly in a wheelchair or in an assisted-living facility, needing help to get dressed and use the bathroom. That's not living; that's existing. In my opinion, there's a huge difference between *quantity* and *quality* of life. It's the difference between *deficient survival* (a term I first heard used by Dr. Robert Heaney at Creighton University) and *exceptional survival*.

Lifestyle Trumps Genetics

How can you square off the curve? Simple: Embrace healthy habits, today. Adopting the ideas discussed throughout this book will contribute to substantially improved odds of you living a long and healthy life. This includes getting proper exercise, nutrition, sleep, and supplementation; managing your weight and stress; not smoking or using drugs; and having moderate or no alcohol consumption. Practicing these healthy habits can improve both the *quality* and the *quantity* of your life. Is it a guarantee that you will have a longer and better life? Of course not, but the increased odds are hard to argue with.

By the way, none of this is particularly new information. Hippocrates, who was born in 460 BC, said, "Walking is man's best medicine." In 1873, Edward Stanley, the Earl of Derby, proclaimed, "Those who think they have not time for bodily exercise will sooner or later have to find time for illness." Today we know that, from a health perspective, you are what your risk factors say you are.

The term *risk factor* actually originated from the Framingham Heart Study, which started in 1948 with just over 5,200 residents in the Boston suburb of Framingham, Massachusetts. The study population included healthy men and women ages thirty to sixty-two who were closely tracked over their lifetimes, known a longitudinal study. Over the years, the Framingham data confirmed that high blood pressure, elevated cholesterol, and smoking contributed greatly to the development of heart disease. The data also indicated that eating a healthy diet, maintaining an appropriate weight, and practicing regular exercise had a very strong influence on preventing heart disease.

The public health leader Dr. Lester Breslow, who became known as Mr. Public Health, was one of the first researchers to actually document the importance of habits and lifestyle. In 1959, he started the Alameda County (California) Human Population Laboratory. Breslow and his colleagues enrolled 7,000 county residents in a study to determine whether they adhered to seven healthy habits. Six of the habits had been identified in previous research: practicing regular exercise, getting regular sleep, not smoking, drinking moderately or not at all, eating regular meals and not snacking in between, and maintaining a normal weight. The seventh habit was eating a regular breakfast, which Dr. Breslow later admitted was just a hunch (and recently has been shown to not necessarily have a significant impact on health, especially as it relates to weight management).

The results of the study, which became available in the early 1970s, showed that a forty-five-year-old who embraced at least six of the seven habits had a life expectancy eleven years longer than an individual who practiced fewer than four of the habits. Possibly even more impressive was the fact that a sixty-year-old who practiced all seven of the habits was as healthy as a thirty-year-old who followed two or fewer. Clearly, lifestyle (habits plus environment) trumps genetics.

The Cooper Clinic Longitudinal Study

The Cooper Clinic Longitudinal Study (CCLS) began in 1970. With the permission of Cooper Clinic patients, their "de-identified" data is transferred to the nonprofit Cooper Research Institute, and that database is the largest of its type in the world, with more than 1.3 million "person-years" of objective data leading to the publication of more than 600 scientific papers. Data from the CCLS contributed greatly to the public-health recommendation of 150 minutes per week of moderate physical activity.

CCLS researchers are currently investigating the relationship between fitness and healthy aging, as well as cost. So far, they've learned that if you are fit in your fifties, you double your odds of living to at least eighty-five. Conversely, if you are not fit in your fifties, your projected lifespan is eight years shorter than if you are fit. From a cost standpoint, preliminary evaluation shows that being fit in midlife lowers Medicare expenses at age eighty by 34 percent for men and 38 percent for women. That's across multiple disease states, including heart disease, stroke, chronic lung disease, chronic kidney disease, diabetes, and Alzheimer's.

The takeaway is pretty simple: You can't change your parents (your genetics), but you have total control over your habits (lifestyle choices). If you embrace a healthy way of living, you will not only substantially increase your odds of living longer, (between six and eleven years longer) but also dramatically increase your odds of pushing back the onset of disability. In essence, that's the *quality* of your life. If you can develop and maintain healthy habits by midlife, you can delay disability by between thirteen and twenty years. That's amazing! *It's never too late to start!*

Think about what you like to do more than anything else—travel, golf, garden, play with (not just watch) your kids or grandkids, ride a bike, climb a mountain, go bowling, whatever your passion might be. Whatever really excites you, think about the possibility of doing that for up to twenty years longer. How great would that be?

My Dad's Story

Watching what happened to my parents had an enormous impact on the way I live my life today. I was adopted, so I don't know much about my birth parents, but the folks who adopted me, whom I view as my mom and dad, certainly were not able to square off the curve. My dad was raised in Jonesboro, a small town outside of Waco, Texas. (If you're old enough, think Mayberry.) From the time he was a little boy, he wanted to fly airplanes. He attended Southern Methodist University in Dallas for a short time, but right after World War II, he joined the US Navy and flew the airlift out of Frankfurt, Germany. After he left the military, he went to work for Pioneer Airlines, which later was gobbled up by Continental Airlines. I was four when my dad was transferred from

El Paso to Los Angeles, and from the time I can remember, I knew that my dad *loved* to fly. It was never a job to him. Without a doubt, it was his *passion*. He was meant to fly. My dad lit up whenever he put on his uniform.

During my freshman year at the University of California–Los Angeles, shortly after my dad was promoted to captain, the professional pinnacle for pilots, he went in for his annual FAA physical—something all commercial pilots are required to do. During a routine stress test on the treadmill, the doctor stopped the exam after just a few minutes. "Why?" my dad asked. "I feel fine."

The doctor's response was a surprise, certainly something he did not expect to hear: "Your test is abnormal. I believe you have heart disease." My dad was shocked. Even though he was a smoker and drank more than he should, was overweight, and fairly inactive, he still "felt fine." A few days later, my father lost his pilot's license. He was devastated that he had been grounded.

In an effort to regain his flying status, my dad went into a full-court press. He attended a thirty-day in-residence lifestyle-modification program; he stopped smoking, lost weight, and started walking regularly. He basically did a 180-degree turn in terms of his lifestyle. He improved his health, but he would never fly again, because the FAA still did not consider it safe for him to pilot a plane. Psychologically, my dad was never the same. They had taken away his passion, the one thing that truly gave him a sense of worth. From the time he lost his license, he lived another seventeen years, though "lived" is not very accurate. He was *alive* for seventeen more years. He had a series of heart operations, (coronary bypass, stents) but ultimately developed congestive heart failure.

I vividly remember one time when I went to see my father at Greene Hospital in La Jolla, California. He was suffering from congestive obstructive pulmonary disorder and could only whisper. He motioned for me to come close. "If you ever let Lauren and Andrew smoke," he said in a faint voice, "it will be the biggest mistake you ever make." He knew that smoking and other poor lifestyle choices had put him where he was.

When my dad was young, no one had known that smoking was bad; it was actually *promoted* in the military. And no one understood that being a couch potato had negative consequences or that eating chicken-fried steak the size of a hubcap would ultimately be detrimental. My dad was from Texas, for cryin' out loud; that's what you did back then! He was seventy when he died.

Mom's Turn

In my senior year at UCLA, I took a ten-week class called The Biology of Cancer. It wasn't a required course, but I didn't know much about cancer and I was interested in the topic. In my sixth week of the class, on Mother's Day, my mom, who was fifty-five at the time, woke up with intense pain in the front part of her right thigh. She was rushed to Torrance (California) Memorial Hospital in an ambulance and was quickly admitted. Doctors thought the pain was caused by some sort of pressure on her sciatic nerve, so they placed her in traction for a week.

Despite the bed rest, she experienced no relief from the pain, which was getting worse. The doctors finally ordered a CAT scan and discovered that my mother had ovarian cancer—a tumor the size of a grapefruit on her right ovary. Stage 3-B, not at all an encouraging diagnosis. It was devastating!

After surgery, my mom had three agonizing weeklong sessions of chemotherapy. The chemo took an extreme toll. She would vomit violently, and lost all of her hair. When she was finally able to regain a modicum of strength, she began a six-week series of radiation treatments. Again, it was no walk in the park. All the while, my mother did her best to keep an optimistic outlook, although she knew the odds, and they weren't good: Ovarian cancer is very aggressive, and the big C could return at any time. For a while, she got better and tried to resume a normal life, but three years later, the cancer came back. She had another surgery, followed by more chemo and more radiation.

From the time my mom was diagnosed to the time she passed away was just over five years. She was sixty-one when she died. Like my dad, my mom had not lived a very healthy lifestyle. She, too, had smoked, although she had finally quit in her forties, was obese, and was almost completely inactive. Before her trip to the hospital on Mother's Day, she had not been to the doctor—any doctor—in more than five years.

I really wish I had known then what I know now. Although my parents both died prematurely, what I remember most is the devastating final years of their lives, in the *deficient survival* category: alive but not living. My parents had a constant fear that their time was extremely limited and, as it turned out, they were right. My children never met my mom, unfortunately, and they were too young to remember my dad.

Looking Downfield

Watching how my parents closed out their lives had a tremendous impact on me. We are all on this earth for a fixed amount of time, but I intend to do everything possible to square off the curve! I don't want just to *watch* the game; I want to be *in* the game! Carve out some time and think about the things that are most important to you. Write them down. What's your future look like? What are your big hairy audacious goals? I can promise, whatever they are, they will be much more achievable if you are healthy and not compromised by poor health.

Take advantage of this wonderful life you've been blessed with. Yes, I know that today's environment is tempting, that physical activity has become optional and that great-tasting, cheap, convenient food is essentially everywhere. It's hard to be healthy—sometimes *really* hard—but I guarantee it's possible. More important, it's worth it!

"History will be kind to me because I plan to write it."
– Winston Churchill

> "Climb the mountain so you can see the world,
> not so the world can see you."

33.

Yeah, Right!

"This will be the hardest thing you'll ever do." That's what I remember most from the large packet of information I received from the trekking company we had hired to help us climb Mt. Kilimanjaro in Tanzania. I thought, *Yeah, right!* Despite the fact that the mountain has an elevation greater than 19,000 feet, I knew Kili was not a technical climb. In my mind, it was just a really long hike. How hard could that be? I mean, come on! I had run four marathons and several half-marathons and sprint triathlons, as well as climbed multiple peaks, including Mt. Whitney, in California, the highest peak in the continental United States, at 14,505 feet. How much tougher could Kilimanjaro be? I was about to find out.

In 2013, my son, Andrew, was getting ready to graduate from college. As he had begun his final year, we had started talking about doing something significant to celebrate his accomplishment. Sam, my buddy since first grade, had suggested we climb Kilimanjaro. I had run it by Drew, and before we knew it, we were making plans to scale the highest peak in Africa. Our climbing party would include Andrew and me; his cousin Michael, who was also graduating from college in California; Sam; and Sam's son, Blake, and daughter, Brooklin—two dads in their late fifties along with four twenty-somethings . . . all four of whom happened to be in terrific shape. Oh, and I should mention, we would also have three guides and twenty-nine—yes, twenty-nine porters! That should have been a clue as to what we had in store!

Although Tanzania is pretty warm year-round, that's not the case when you get above about 12,000 feet. A bit of research told us that June was the warmest and driest month at the top of Kili, which is actually a volcano that rises dramatically from the African desert high into the clouds. It even has its own weather system, and snow at the top year-round. The timing worked out perfectly with Drew's graduation which, was scheduled for May. Because he and I were in Dallas and the four others were in Southern California, the plan was for us to all meet up in Amsterdam, then fly together the nine or so hours to the small airport not far from the mountain.

The flight Andrew and I took into Amsterdam was on time, but the connection for the others was delayed, so Drew and I had a free day in the city of Moshi before the others could catch up. Talk about a cultural whiplash! It's one thing to read and hear about the challenging circumstances in most of Africa, but it's quite another to experience it firsthand. It sounds trite, but compared to most of the world, we have so much to be thankful for! Moshi is a big city, with almost 200,000 residents, but it was a far, far departure from the type of communities we have in America. Our trekking company had arranged for clean and secure accommodations, but virtually everywhere we turned, we saw abject poverty. Although most everyone was friendly, we stuck out like sore thumbs, and we had to constantly keep moving to avoid being engulfed by spirited teams of beggars and artisans.

The California contingent made it to Moshi the next day, and we began preparing for our trek. We met our guides, packed our gear, and learned specifically what to expect. Although there are six official routes up the mountain, they all lead to the same place, and that place is high—specifically, 19,340 feet high. I still really had no clue what that meant, as I had never been above 15,000 feet, but much of our orientation dealt with the topic of altitude and what to do if something went wrong. I was nervously comforted by the fact that, at all times, one of our porters, Matote, would be within just a few feet of us with a portable inflatable hyperbaric chamber. If anyone were to be struck by altitude sickness, which is rather common, the support team would immediately inflate the chamber, place the person inside, and then carry that person off the mountain. It's known as medical evacuation. Reassuring, yes?

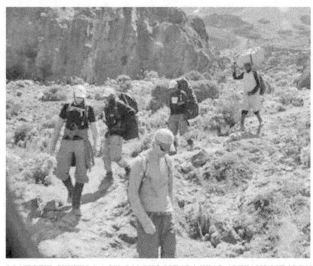

MATOTE (WITH PACK ON HIS HEAD) WAS ALWAYS NEARBY
IF ANYTHING HAD GONE WRONG

The next morning, we loaded up in a van and took off on a two-hour ride to the base of the mountain. Andrew and I had been in Africa for more than two days by then, and we still had not actually *seen* Kilimanjaro. It had, rather eerily, been constantly shrouded by thick, billowy clouds.

By the way, if you think folks in New York or L.A. drive crazy, it doesn't compare to the daredevils on the roads in Africa! There are cars, trucks, vans, buses, scooters, and motorcycles—hundreds and hundreds of motorcycles—all trying to get somewhere else, in a hurry. Once we were out of the city, a guy on a motorcycle tried to pass our van and was clipped by the side mirror of a truck coming the other way. BAM! It happened right beside us, right there! With an enormous thud, the motorcyclist caromed off the side of our van and was thrown into a ditch. We immediately pulled over. He was not moving, and we were pretty convinced he was dead. Fortunately, we were wrong. After a few minutes, he came to, and it was clear his biggest concern was not *his* condition but *his bike's* condition, as it was probably his only means of making a living. There were a ton of folks shouting in Swahili, so we never really got the whole picture, but after about fifteen minutes, we were back on our way.

After entering Kilimanjaro National Park, our guides began the process of selecting porters. Several dozen candidates, all male, gathered in the hopes of being selected for a climb, which usually takes somewhere between five and eleven days. Being a porter is exceptionally hard work because porters must carry heavy, bulky equipment and supplies up a mountain—and do it quickly. The porters' job is to have that night's camp completely ready—i.e., tents and temporary bathrooms set up, water available, and meals nearly prepared—by the time the hiking party makes it there by midafternoon. Most porters hope to make two or three climbs per month in order to properly support their families. They are all, to no surprise, incredibly fit, and apparently amazingly happy, despite the challenges. (Whenever I find myself frustrated with my "day job," I think about the life of a porter and my pity party comes to a grinding halt really quick!)

The actual climb of Kili is fascinating, as you experience five ecosystems along the way. We started in a rain forest, and before long, we were, as I can best describe it, in a jungle. It was pretty hot, very muggy, and awfully muddy. Our guides continually implored us to "polepole!" (pronounced "Paulie Paulie"—Swahili for "slow down"). Even though we were still well below 10,000 feet, I suspect this was primarily to get us accustomed to taking our time and to prepare us for the latter parts of the ascent, when there would be less and less air with each and every step.

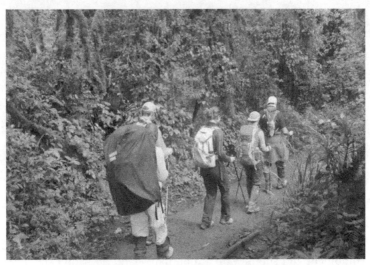

JUST STARTING OUT IN THE RAIN FOREST

It's a bit difficult to get accurate updated statistics, but only about 65 percent of those who attempt to climb Kilimanjaro actually make it to the summit. Most folks fail because they don't respect the power of altitude. It's possible to reach the peak in three or four days, but your odds of success go way up if you allow yourself to gradually acclimate over the course of several days. Altitude couldn't care less about your experience, education, or fitness level; if you don't respect her, she will make you pay a hefty price. We had opted for a nine-day climb (seven up and two down), which seemed to be the formula most likely to produce a successful summit. I've long been a believer that success leaves clues, and since our guides did this for a living, I was determined to be extremely coachable, so *polepole* it was! I was not going to travel halfway around the world and not reach the top of that darned mountain . . . even though I still had not even seen it!

When we made it to camp by mid-afternoon of our first day, everything was set. Our tents were up, with our gear placed neatly inside. We were tired but not whipped. I suspect that my adrenaline level was somewhat elevated in anticipation of what was coming over the next several days. We had been planning this expedition for months, but now it was real: We were actually camping at the base of the largest free-standing mountain in the world! If all went according to plan, in six days, we would reach the peak!

That night, we had dinner in a large tent that accommodated all six of us. The food was fantastic. One thing I quickly noticed was that when the sun went down, so did the temperature—almost instantly! It seemed to happen as if someone had flipped a switch. Temperatures during the day were very comfortable, but at night, they dropped well below freezing. We slept in fairly small two-man tents; I bunked with Drew, Sam with Brooklin, and Mike with Blake. We had excellent sleeping bags rated for sub-freezing environments, but it was still *very cold*! And because we were hyper-intentional about staying hydrated, getting up at night to pee was always a large physical and psychological hurdle. That first night was not very restful.

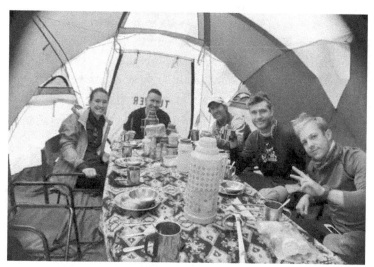

"CHOW TIME!"

"Do . . . do" was our guides' greeting to wake us up the next morning, and every morning thereafter. We never got an exact translation, but it was basically a gentle encouragement to "get your butt out of bed." As we slowly made our way out of our tents, there was already a buzz of activity. The guides and porters were busy prepping for the day's climb; they seemed excited. Everyone greeted us with an energetic "Jambo!" (hello!), and they even broke into a rousing chorus of "Hakuna Matata" (No Worries!... remember *The Lion King*?) before we broke camp. It was awesome. It was also obvious "we weren't in Kansas" anymore!

After some tea and a hearty breakfast, we took off. We were still very much in the rain forest, and not until late morning did we rise above what I would describe as the tree line and transition into an arctic desert. At this point, it was wide open, not overly steep, but we still could not see our target. Off in the distance was an enormous cloud; we knew the mountain was underneath it somewhere, but it was hard to get a feel about exactly what we had in front of us. I still vividly remember when, during a short rest, one of the guides pointed at a very specific part of the cloud and said, "If it were a clear day, you would see her *right there*," and then, immediately, as if on cue, the clouds parted and revealed a gigantic isolated, ominous mountain. It could not have been scripted any better, and it was *incredible*! There was no more need to guess about what awaited us. There she was—and she was big . . .very, *very big*! It was then that I realized this was clearly more than just a long hike!

The next five days were very consistent: wake up, eat breakfast, have our vital signs (pulse, oxygen saturation, etc.) checked, break camp, hike for two or three hours, stop for a sack lunch, have vitals checked again, hike another few hours, get to camp by midafternoon, clean up as best we could (we obviously had no showers but did have, thanks to the porters, clean water), maybe take a nap, eat dinner, check our vital signs once more, discuss the next day's agenda with the guides, then head to bed pretty early.

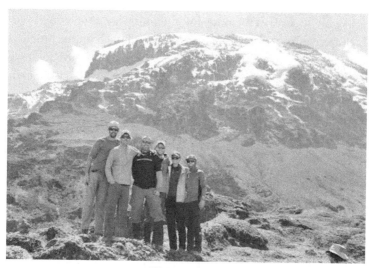

"THAT'S HER!"

The only variance was that with every new day, the trail became steeper and each night we were camping at an elevation that was usually higher than the night before. We certainly weren't the only group on the mountain, but for the most part, other than at the campgrounds, we didn't see many other parties. There was zero communication with the rest of the world—obviously no cell phones, no newspapers, no Internet, and no radio or TV. To be honest, it was rather refreshing.

Our guides were all very pleasant and had playful personalities, but one thing they took very seriously was our health. They were all medically trained and kept a very close watch on our physical conditions. I'm sure part of their evaluation was how many of their hikers actually got to the top safely, so it gave me confidence that they were so adamant about not pushing the envelope at any point during our journey.

The natural rhythm of the hikes allowed for a rotation so two or three of us would fall in line with one another and have conversations about all sorts so things. Sometimes, though, we just walked in silence. At the time, I was seriously contemplating a very big career shift, so Sam and I talked a great deal about the pros and cons of such a move. (I later made the change and have jokingly said the decision was actually made at very high altitude in extremely thin air!)

Nights on the mountain were both beautiful and tough. Often, we were *above* the clouds. The sky was crystal clear, and the stars seemed to be almost within reach. As you might expect, it was very, very quiet. The big challenge, though, besides the cold temps, was that, as we made our way up the mountain, it was hard to find flat terrain. It was tough for me to get comfortable while sleeping at an angle, so the fatigue factor really began to build after the first couple days.

One thing in particular that I found impressive was the way Brooklin handled everything. I've known "Brookie" since almost the day she was born, so I had suspected she would do great, but I was blown away with how well she adapted to the very trying circumstances. Besides the physical nature of the hike, she was the only female in our group of six, surrounded by thirty-two men (three guides plus twenty-nine porters), most of whom spoke little to no English. While hiking, when nature called for us dudes, it was no big deal to make a quick detour, but it wasn't nearly as simple for Brooklin. Never, not even once, did I hear Brooklin utter a complaint, though. She was the ultimate trooper!

Each and every day, we moved closer to the peak. We were on the Lemosho route, which meant we approached the mountain from the west, then, over the last four days, wrapped around the south side and made the final ascent from the southeast. The night before we summited was spent at Barafu Camp, at an altitude of 14,950 feet. Everyone, including our guides, seemed quieter than normal. By then, everyone was pretty fatigued from six straight days of hiking, but, more importantly, we all recognized that the next day was going to be a bear.

Summit day started at five a.m., earlier than normal. Almost immediately, something felt different. To this point, my appetite

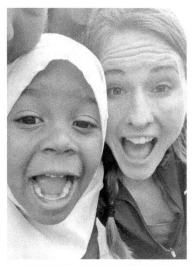

BROOKLIN MAKES A FRIEND

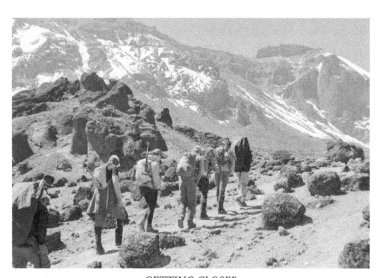

GETTING CLOSER

had been voracious, which was not that unusual. I figured I had been burning at least 6,000 calories per day, so it took plenty of food to keep me fueled. On this morning, though, I had no appetite . . . at all. That *never* happens. I forced myself to eat, but it wasn't nearly the amount I was accustomed to. This, I would find out later, would come back to bite me.

What I remember most about summit day was the very tangible effects of the altitude. The climb was steeper than that of any of the previous days, and it was obvious that with each step, less and less oxygen was available. What's interesting about altitude is that its effect is curvilinear, meaning that the effect of the transition from, say, 8,000 feet to 9,000 feet is not nearly as dramatic as from 18,000 feet to 19,000 feet. I had studied this in school and we had talked about it all week, but on this day, it became extremely real. The best way I can describe it is to imagine walking on a treadmill at a very steep incline while breathing through a wet beach towel. Breathing faster was of little help. We had to constantly focus on taking slow, deep breaths, and never was the concept of "*polepole*" more critical.

The plan was to take six or so hours to reach the crest of the volcano, an area known as Stella Point (elevation 18,471 feet). It was only two miles away from where we started the morning, but it felt as if it were straight up. By this time, we were beginning to get into the arctic snowcap and our path was not quite as "defined" as it had been at the lower altitudes. Now, even though this endeavor had become a significant physical challenge, it was also a big stretch psychologically. It would have been easy to call it quits . . . especially when we occasionally experienced hikers headed down the mountain who looked like death after failing to make it.

What proved to be amazingly helpful was the collective attitude of our team of my five "family" members and our three guides. There was very much a "one for all and all for one" mindset, and I knew that somehow, some way, we were going to find a way for us to all reach the top.

It took a massive effort, but we made it to Stella Point in just over five hours and broke for lunch. The guides checked our vitals, and although a couple of the young climbers needed a bit of supplemental oxygen, there was no doubt we were going to make it. We still had three quarters of a mile to hike to the peak, but the elevation increase was *only* 869 feet (compared to the 3,521feet we had already scaled). I still had almost no appetite, and nothing at all sounded appealing. Even the thought of food made me somewhat nauseous. I *knew* I needed fuel, but I just couldn't bring myself to eat anything. Instead, I made sure I was properly hydrated and figured I'd be fine.

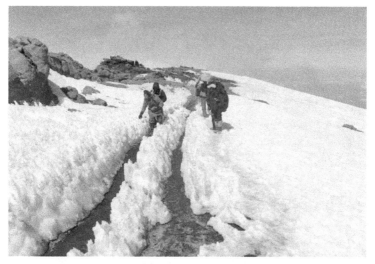

SUMMIT DAY – OH SO CLOSE!

The final push was actually much tougher than I had expected. There was quite a bit of snow on the ground, and the wind, which had been almost nonexistent before this day, began to pick up a bit. It didn't matter, though. We knew we were literally moments away from reaching what we had been planning for months—the top of Mt. Kilimanjaro!

We made it to the summit just after two p.m., and we had the place to ourselves. Some groups start their final climb at midnight so they can reach the peak at sunrise, but we had opted for the additional sleep. I'm glad we did, especially because we could celebrate and take pictures without having to share the area. I must admit that despite being dog tired, I felt an amazing sense of accomplishment. Andrew and I embraced in a father-son hug at "the top of the world," and I was thrilled to share that experience with him and my nephew, Michael. It was also great to "check that box" with Sam and his two kids.

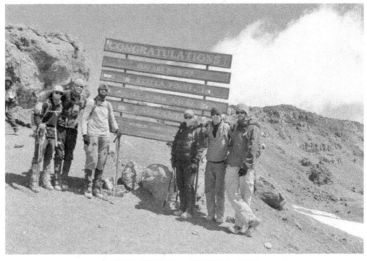

WE MADE IT! - JUNE 27, 2013

After forty or so minutes of high fives and celebration, it was time for us to reverse course. We still had a lot of ground to cover, although working *with* gravity is far easier than working *against* it. We hiked back to Stella Point and stopped for a short break before the descending trek back to Barafu Camp, where we had started the day many hours earlier.

It was during this break that I bonked—a term that endurance athletes often use to describe completely running out of gas. It also is sometimes referred to as hitting the wall. This became glaringly apparent to everyone when I asked if they could see the hang gliders. "The what?" they responded. I countered, "The hang gliders! Look, they're right there!" as I pointed into the distance. Clearly, I was a bit delirious, since there most likely was not a hang glider within 1,000 miles of where we were.

At this point, the guides started to strategize a game plan. My vitals were fine, but I was having a hard time standing up and was not going to make it more than two miles down a steep mountain on my own. It was weird, because the mental fuzziness had gone away pretty quickly, but I still was not very physically stable. I knew exactly what was going on, because I had bonked twice before: one time while training for a marathon and once while running one. It had never been this dramatic, though, and certainly never in such a remote location. Because I had not eaten much that day, I had completely depleted my glycogen (carbohydrate) stores, the primary fuel for the muscles and brain. Our guides quickly started giving me a white powdery mix that they called African cocaine. Don't worry, it was really just pure carbohydrate (sugar), which was exactly what I needed to refuel my system.

The decision was made for one of the guides to go with the "kids" back down to Barafu while the other two guides and Sam took a much slower approach with me. I will forever be grateful for their assistance. I had someone to lean on, mostly Sam, all the way back to camp. I talked almost the entire time, which Sam interpreted as a very positive sign. Historically when I get quiet, it means something is amiss. We arrived long after dark, and even though I felt okay, I was completely exhausted and still was not hungry, so I went straight to bed. It was the best night of sleep I'd had in a week.

The next morning, I woke up and felt great. And guess what? I was famished! After devouring an enormous breakfast, I felt as if nothing had ever been wrong. We were scheduled to take two days to get down to the base of the mountain, but the morning hike went so well that we collectively decided to just go for it. A hot shower and cold beer sounded *really* good, so we covered 9.3 miles in about six hours. There were parts of the hike when we actually ran for a bit.

Sharing this story reinforces what an amazing experience it was for me. It's a long way of demonstrating the importance of *why.* There was no way I could have *bought* what resulted from that trip; I had to *earn* it. I will forever share memories with my son, my nephew, and Sam's family that happened only because we were all fit enough to do it.

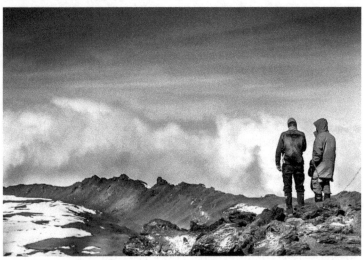

WITH ANDREW AT THE SUMMIT, FOR ME... A PRICELESS PHOTO

Now, I fully recognize that you may have absolutely no interest in climbing Kilimanjaro—or any other mountain, for that matter—but wouldn't it be cool to know that you *could* do it if you had to? I firmly believe that life is better with options—and if you can routinely make investments in yourself, your options are basically unlimited. Your potential is tremendous, and I sincerely hope that you can embrace at least some of the recommendations I have shared so you can live a fantastically fulfilling life . . . and leave the campground cleaner than you found it! Be well!

"There is more in us than we know.
If we can be made to see it, perhaps,
for the rest of our lives we'll be unwilling to settle for less."
– Kurt Hahn

Appendix

Should you decide you'd like to climb Mt. Kilimanjaro, you will need to hire a trekking company. There are many, many options, and I encourage you to really do your homework. Keep in mind that not all operators are created equal and that price is only one of the many factors you need to consider. We used Tusker Trail Adventures out of Lake Tahoe, based on the recommendation of my good friend David Michel. We were very pleased, but there are other trekking companies that have outstanding reputations as well. I encourage you to find an operator who has a commitment to porter welfare and is supportive of organizations such as KPAP (Kilimanjaro Porters Assistance Project).

Since our Kili climb, I have had the amazing fortune of getting to know Dr. Richard Deming, an oncologist based in Des Moines, Iowa. Besides being one of our country's leading medical specialists, Dr. Deming is the founder of Above+Beyond Cancer, a public charity "with a mission to elevate the lives of those touched by cancer, to create a healthier world." If the account of our Kilimanjaro experience has your wheels spinning, then you must explore www.aboveandbeyondcancer.org. Every year, Dr. Deming leads a group of cancer patients, survivors, caregivers, medical experts, and volunteers on what he calls a Gonzo Trip. Besides Kilimanjaro, they've been on adventures to Nepal, Machu Picchu, Everest Base Camp, and the High Himalaya. Each adventure is coupled with some sort of medical mission, and the stories that result are absolutely incredible. Dr. Deming's greatest ambition is to encourage others to pursue lives of meaning, purpose, passion, and compassion. From my perspective, that's one heck of a *why!*

QUOTE SUMMARY
(attributions included where available)

"I don't want to watch my grandkids play. I want to play
with my grandkids."
– Todd Whitthorne

"Good health is not about temporary behavior change.
It's about building healthy habits that will last a lifetime!"
– Todd Whitthorne

"The first step is to establish that something is
possible...then probability will occur."
- Elon Musk

"When the student is ready, the teacher will appear."
- Buddhist Proverb

"You can't live a perfect day without doing something
for someone who will never be able to repay you."
- John Wooden

"We need to leave the campground cleaner
than we found it!"
- George Bein

"The human body is beautifully designed. It will do whatever you ask it to do."
- Todd Whitthorne

"Take the first step in faith. You don't have to see the
whole staircase, just take the first step."
- Dr. Martin Luther King, Jr.

"Knowing is not enough; we must apply. Wishing is not enough; we must do."
- Johann Von Goethe

"Yes, there are two paths you can go by, but in the long run there's still time to change the road you're on."
- Stairway to Heaven, Led Zeppelin

"Do not fear failure. Fear average."

"You are what your record says you are."
- Bill Parcells

"The time to repair the roof is when the sun is shining."
- John F. Kennedy

"If you do not change direction you may end up where you are heading."
- Lao Tzu

"If you've got your health you're a zillionaire."
- Dick Vitale

"We should all be concerned with the future because we're going to spend the rest of our lives there."
- Charles F. Kettering

"If we did all the things we are capable of we would literally, astound ourselves."
- Thomas Edison

"A wise man proportions his belief to the evidence."
- David Hume

"I can't believe that God put us on this earth to be ordinary."
- Lou Holtz

"What saves a man is to take a step.
Then another step. It is always the same step,
but you have to take it."
- Antoine de-Saint Exupery

"Yes, exercise is the catalyst. That's what makes
everything happen: your digestion, your elimination, your
sex life, your skin, hair, everything about you depends on
circulation. And how do you increase circulation?"
- Jack LaLanne

"Without ambition, one starts nothing.
Without work, one finishes nothing.
The prize will not be sent to you. You have to win it."
- Ralph Waldo Emerson

"You will never change your life until you change
something you do daily."
- Mike Murdoch

"Success is the sum of small efforts repeated day in and
day out."
- Robert Collier

"A small daily task, if it be really daily,
will beat the labours of a spasmodic Hercules."
- Anthony Trollope

"Our body is a machine for living.
It is organized for that, it is its nature."
- Leo Tolstoy

"Eat food, not too much, mostly plants."
- Michael Pollan

"Man is what he eats."
- Ludwig Feuerbach

"Never give up on something that you can't go a day without thinking about."
- Winston Churchill

"Hara hachi bu…(Eat until you are 80% full.")
- Confucius

"Don't be afraid to go out on a limb. That's where the fruit is."
- H. Jackson Browne

"Avoid fried foods, which angry up the blood."
- Satchel Paige

"As a child, my family's menu consisted of two choices: take it, or leave it."
- Buddy Hackett

"Ask yourself what is really important and then have the courage to build your life around the answer."

"If a million people say a foolish thing, it is still a foolish thing."
- Anatole France

"Truth is not diminished by the number of people that believe it."

"If you have a body, you're an athlete."
- Bill Bowerman

"Life is like a ten-speed bicycle. Most of us have gears we never use."
- Charles Schultz

"If you had to pick one thing to make people healthier as they age, it would be aerobic exercise."
- Dr. James Fries

"Your priorities are defined by what you do, not by what you say."
– Todd Whitthorne

"A man's health can be judged by which he takes two at a time...pills or stairs."
- Joan Welsh

"Those who think they have not time for bodily exercise will sooner or later have to find time for illness."
- Edward Stanley

"The doctor of the future will give no medicine, but will invest his patients in the care of the human frame, in diet and in the cause and prevention of disease."
- Thomas Edison

"We don't stop playing because we grow old; we grow old because we stop playing."
- George Bernard Shaw

"The elevator to success is out of order.
You'll have to use the stairs...one at a time."
- Joe Girard

"To give anything less than your best,
is to sacrifice the gift."
- Steve Prefontaine

"Walk the dog, even if you don't have one."
– Todd Whitthorne

"Life is like riding a bicycle.
You don't fall off unless you stop pedaling."
- Claude D. Pepper

"If you are not making someone's life better,
you are wasting your time."

"You must be present to win."
- Bill Case

"Knowing your sense of purpose is worth up to seven
years of extra life expectancy."
- Dan Buettner

"Whoever I am or whatever I am doing, some kind of
excellence is within my reach."
- John W. Gardner

"If you don't like where you are, move.
You are not a tree."

"Motivation is what gets you going. Habit is what keeps you going."
– Jim Rohn

"We are what we repeatedly do.
Excellence then, is not an act, but a habit."
- Aristotle

"You learn much more from your failures than you do from success."
- Todd Whitthorne

"The direction you are headed in is much more important than your velocity."

"Success leaves clues."
– Tony Robbins

"Turn a bad day into good data."
– Ron McMillan

"Health is a journey, not a destination."
- Todd Whitthorne

"The choices we make are a function
of the choices we have."
- Dr. David Katz

"A year from now you will wish you had started today."

"You drown not by falling into a river,
but by staying submerged in it."
- Paulo Cuelho

"It's not what happens to you that's important, it's how you handle what happens to you."
- Todd Whitthorne

"Don't let mental blocks control you. Set yourself free. Confront your fear and turn the mental blocks into building blocks."
- Roopleen

"When you bow, bow low."
- Asian motto as relayed by Dr. Stephen Covey

"You'll never leave where you are until you decide where you'd rather be."

"If you keep doing what you've been doing, you'll keep getting what you've been getting."
- Zig Ziglar

"If it's important to you, you'll find a way. If it's not, you'll find an excuse."

"Finish each day & be done with it. You have done what you could. Learn from it; tomorrow is a new day."
- Ralph Waldo Emerson

"Age is a case of mind over matter. If you don't mind, it don't matter."
- Satchel Paige

"Live your life and forget your age."
– Norman Vincent Peale

"The benefit of vitamin D is as clear as the harmful link between smoking and lung cancer."
- Dr. Cedrick Garland

"Sunlight might prevent thirty deaths for each one caused by skin cancer."
– Dr. Edward Giovannucci

"Eat fish, not hotdogs."
- Dr. Joseph Hibbeln

"If it came from a plant, eat it.
If it was made in a plant don't."
- Michael Pollan

"An army marches on its stomach."
- Napolean Bonaparte

"Success is piece of mind which is a direct result of knowing you did your best to become the best you are capable of becoming."
- John Wooden

"People often say that motivation doesn't last. Well, neither does bathing – that's why we recommend it daily."
- Zig Ziglar

"We know nothing about motivation.
We just write books about it."
- Peter Drucker

"For a habit to stay changed, people must believe change is possible and most often, that belief only emerges with the help of a group."
– Charles Duhigg

"Impossible is not a fact, it's an opinion."

"The entire population of the universe, with one trifling exception, is composed of others."
- John Andrew Holmes

"Don't trip over things behind you."

"It always seems impossible until it's done."
- Nelson Mandela

"The power of one, if fearless and focused, is formidable, but the power of many working together is better."
- Gloria Macapagal Arroyo

"A human being is happiest and most successful when dedicated to a cause outside his own individual selfish satisfaction."
- Dr. Benjamin Spock

"Do or do not. There is no try."
- Yoda

"One person can make a difference. Be that person."
- Wyland

"If you ask me what I came into this life to do, I will tell you: I came to live out loud."
- Emile Zola

"Walking is man's best medicine."
- Hippocrates

"History will be kind to me because I plan to write it."
- Winston Churchill

"Climb the mountain so you can see the world, not so the world can see you."

"There is more in us than we know.
If we can be made to see it, perhaps,
for the rest of our lives we'll be unwilling to settle for less."
- Kurt Hahn

"If diamonds were as plentiful as grains of sand they would be worthless. If we lived forever, wasting a day of our lives would be trivial. But it's precisely the fact that we don't live forever that makes today so valuable. So what are you going to do with your life today?
- Dr. Richard Deming